CARE SKILLS
FOR NURSES

Student Survival Skills Series

Survive your nursing course with these essential guides for all student nurses:

Calculation Skills for Nurses
Claire Boyd
9781118448892

Medicine Management Skills for Nurses
Claire Boyd
9781118448854

Clinical Skills for Nurses
Claire Boyd
9781118448779

Care Skills for Nurses
Claire Boyd
9781118657386

CARE SKILLS
FOR NURSES

Claire Boyd
RGN, Cert Ed
Practice Development Trainer

WILEY Blackwell

This edition first published 2014
© 2014 by John Wiley & Sons, Ltd

Registered office:
John Wiley & Sons, Ltd, The Atrium, Southern Gate, Chichester, West Sussex, PO19 8SQ, UK

Editorial offices:
9600 Garsington Road, Oxford, OX4 2DQ, UK
The Atrium, Southern Gate, Chichester, West Sussex, PO19 8SQ, UK
111 River Street, Hoboken, NJ 07030-5774, USA

For details of our global editorial offices, for customer services and for information about how to apply for permission to reuse the copyright material in this book please see our website at www.wiley.com/wiley-blackwell

Library of Congress Cataloging-in-Publication Data
Boyd, Claire, author.
  Care skills for nurses / Claire Boyd.
      p. ; cm. – (Student survival skills series)
  Includes bibliographical references and index.
  ISBN 978-1-118-65738-6 (pbk. : alk. paper) – ISBN 978-1-118-65734-8 (mobi) – ISBN 978-1-118-65736-2
(epub) – ISBN 978-1-118-65737-9 (epdf) – ISBN 978-1-118-75738-3 – ISBN 978-1-118-75766-6
  I. Title.   II. Series: Student survival skills series.
  [DNLM: 1. Nursing Care–methods–Handbooks. WY 49]
  RT41
  610.73–dc23
                                                                                            2013024791

A catalogue record for this book is available from the British Library.

Wiley also publishes its books in a variety of electronic formats. Some content that appears in print may not be available in electronic books.

Cover image courtesy of Visual Philosophy
Chapter opener image: © iStockphoto.com/kokouu
Cover design by Visual Philosophy

1   2014

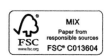

Contents

Preface

This book is designed to assist the student healthcare worker in 12 aspects of nursing that may be utilised in the hospital or community setting. It is designed to give a quick, snappy introduction to these skills in a non-threatening manner, allowing the reader to gain a brief understanding and overview. The aim is then to build on these skills.

Care and compassion are the two central themes running through this book, and due to their importance in the healthcare environment they are also the subject of the first chapter, which emphasises the importance of these key skills.

The book talks about 'patients' but often uses the community terminology of 'service user' as well. The paediatric nurse has not been forgotten, with information throughout incorporating this branch of nursing.

The book incorporates many exercises to check understanding, and is presented in a simple to follow step-by-step approach, ending with Test Your Knowledge exercises to relate learning to practice. The aim of this book is to start the individual on a journey through many healthcare-related exercises to help build confidence and competence: from day one to qualification, and beyond.

It has been compiled by quotes and tips from student nurses themselves: it is a book by students for students.

Claire Boyd
Bristol
May 2013

Preface

Introduction

Hello, my name is Claire and I am a Practice Development Trainer in a large NHS trust. I began my nurse training many years ago now, but still remember my first day 'on the wards' and how scary it felt. In my very first placement I was sent to the neighbouring ward for 'a long stand'. Thinking this was some sort of medical equipment, I duly obliged. I asked for the long stand and then waited, and waited, and waited, before realising I had been 'had' and the brunt of my new co-worker's joke. It seems that with increasing workloads many of us have lost our sense of humour, and according to recent press reports our 'capacity to care'.

In my time as a nurse, if I was caring for a patient with a specific medical condition that I did not understand I would go to the university library to collect a book on the subject: no worldwide web at that time! Many of these books were informative, but they were too large and went into too much detail; in short, they were far too in-depth. I wanted a book I could carry around with me, to 'dip into', to gather the basic facts.

How I would have liked a small, snappy and clearly written book to help me to gain the information I needed, on the topics that I wanted to know about, enabling me to build my understanding. It is worth remembering, however, that although books can give the theory, the care aspect of nursing comes from within.

This book contains common nursing care activities that you may be required to perform, giving you the basics for use in your clinical placements. It treats those we are giving the care to – the patients and service users – in a holistic, compassionate and caring manner.

Some of these nursing care skills will require further training, supervision and/or proof of competence before being 'let loose'. For example, taking an ECG recording will require training to use the ECG machine, and supervision will be required before conducting a bowel assessment.

You may be required to weigh your patient, on admission or as part of their ongoing care, so a weight conversion chart has been provided as Appendix 2 at the end of the book.

Lastly, you will come across many terms that may seem alien to you. Sitting through some handovers can feel like you are in a foreign language class! Many clinical placement areas have orientation packs for new staff, with a list of the most common terms used in that area. It is also always worth purchasing a nursing dictionary for understanding and never to be afraid to ask questions if you don't know something. Many medical words and terms can be more readily understood if you become familiar with prefixes, suffixes and combining forms. With these components it is often possible to work out the meaning of new words. Appendix 1 lists some of these components and their meaning.

Good caring. Remember that it is our privilege to care for our patients and that it takes a *remarkable person to be a nurse.*

Acknowledgements

First acknowledgements go to the student nurses who have made this book possible with their hints and tips, which they have shared for those following in their footsteps.

Acknowledgements also go to North Bristol NHS Trust and specifically Jane Hadfield (Head of Learning and Development) and all my friends and colleagues in the Staff Development Department.

Thanks also to Magenta Styles (Executive Editor of Wiley Blackwell) for first approaching me about this exciting project, Madeleine Hurd (Associate Commissioning Editor), Catriona Cooper (Project Editor) and to freelance editor Nik Prowse for copy-editing the text for me.

I thank Dansac Limited for allowing the reproduction of the images of stoma products in Chapter 7, the Royal College of Nursing for permission to use the Principles of Nursing Practice in Chapter 1 and the Resuscitation Council (UK).

This book is dedicated to my loving family: my long-suffering husband Rob, my Rock (thanks also for the photographs), and Simon and Louise and David. Thank you for all your support.

Chapter 1

CARE AND COMPASSION IN NURSING

Care Skills for Nurses, First Edition. Claire Boyd
© 2014 John Wiley & Sons, Ltd. Published 2014 by John Wiley & Sons, Ltd.

LEARNING OUTCOMES

By the end of this chapter you will have an understanding of the meaning of care and compassion in nursing.

The reasons that individuals cite for wanting to work in the healthcare setting are numerous and varied. Personally, I went into nursing because I wanted to do some good: to help people. The biggest compliment I was ever paid in my nursing career was when a relative visiting her father told me that she wanted to go into nursing after watching me work on the ward and wanted to be 'just like you – kind and caring'. However, visiting the wards in many different hospitals, and in community care homes, it seems that 'kindness' may often be in short supply.

It is true that nursing has been through many changes: not always all for the good. We have all seen the headlines citing lapses in basic care and how today's nurses 'have lost their compassion'. It seems that nursing is receiving a bad press at present and, although it shames me to say this, it is not always unjustified. This has prompted the Royal College of Nursing to launch a campaign, This is Nursing, to show the 'skill and compassion' of today's nurses, as well as to explore the reasons behind failures in care (Royal College of Nursing 2012). This campaign, developed jointly by the Royal College of Nursing, the Nursing and Midwifery Council and the Department of Health, has produced the Principles of Nursing Practice (Royal College of Nursing 2010), which tell us what patients, colleagues, families and carers can expect from nursing. These principles are reproduced in Table 1.1.

The Department of Health and the NHS Commissioning Board (2012) have developed a consultation/discussion paper entitled 'Developing the culture of compassionate care: creating a new vision for nurses, midwives and care-givers' to emphasise values and behaviours that apply in the NHS, public health and social care (Box 1.1).

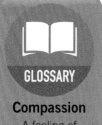

GLOSSARY

Compassion
A feeling of distress and pity for the suffering or misfortune of others. This often includes the desire to alleviate it.

Table 1.1 The Principles of Nursing Practice

A	Nurses and nursing staff treat everyone in their care with dignity and humanity – they understand their individual needs, show compassion and sensitivity, and provide care in a way that respects all people equally.
B	Nurses and nursing staff take responsibility for the care they provide and answer for their own judgements and actions – they carry out these actions in a way that is agreed with their patients, and their families and carers of their patients, and in a way that meets the requirements of their professional bodies and the law.
C	Nurses and nursing staff manage risk, are vigilant about risk, and help to keep everyone safe in the places they receive health care.
D	Nurses and nursing staff provide and promote care that puts people at the centre, involves patients, service users, their families and their carers in decisions and helps them make informed choices about their treatment and care.
E	Nurses and nursing staff are at the heart of the communication process: they assess, record and report on treatment and care, handle information sensitively and confidentially, deal with complaints effectively, and are conscientious in reporting the things they are concerned about.
F	Nurses and nursing staff have an up-to-date knowledge and skills, and use these with intelligence, insight and understanding in line with the needs of each individual in their care.
G	Nurses and nursing staff work closely with their own team and with other professionals, making sure patients' care and treatment is co-ordinated, is of a high standard and has the best possible outcome.
H	Nurses and nursing staff lead by example, develop themselves and other staff, and influence the way care is given in a manner that is open and responds to individual needs.

Permission kindly agreed by Royal College of Nursing. From Royal College of Nursing (2010).

Box 1.1   Culture of compassionate care

Care
Compassion
Competence
Communication
Courage
Commitment

Source: Department of Health and NHS Commissioning Board (2012).

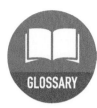

GLOSSARY

Steroid-induced psychosis
A common side effect of the use of any corticosteroid, such as prednisolone. An individual may experience feelings of elation, euphoria and/or extreme mania, delusions of grandeur, hallucinations, general disorientation or psychotic behaviour.

In short, we need to pull our socks up and get back to the basics. Care and compassion are the two central themes of this book. Personally I do not believe that compassion can be taught, but there may be times when we should be reminded of this central ethos and the privileged position that we have when caring for others. I do believe firmly, however, that care and compassion still exist in the healthcare setting, but that they may need a bit of prompting to show themselves; hence the Department of Health, Royal College of Nursing and Nursing and Midwifery Council initiatives.

Always remember: it could be us on the receiving end of care, or one of our loved ones. How would we like to be treated and how would we like our loved ones to be treated? I have been privileged to care for many wonderful people, ranging from those new to the world to those taking their very last breath. For all my patients and service users (people cared for in the community setting) I always strived to provide the very best care with kindness, care and compassion.

Now, let's remove the rose-tinted glasses: some patients may be difficult to care for; they may be confused, frightened or aggressive due to their medical condition. They may be 'under the influence' of drugs or drink and not acting rationally. I've had chairs thrown at me due to 'steroid-induced psychosis' and there were times when I had to remember that my patient was 'ill'. Some patients may just be naturally aggressive, but all patients must be treated with respect and dignity.

Let's look at the case study in Activity 1.1. How much care and compassion has been shown to this patient?

In 2011 The Patients Association (a charitable organisation that aims to tackle poor care and its causes; www.patients-association.com) published a report entitled 'We've been listening, have you been learning?'. It gave the most common complaints received by The Patients Association from patients.

Activity 1.1
Care and compassion exercise

Sarah Matthews was admitted to your clinical area this morning after falling down the stairs. She requires metal fixation surgery to her right tibia and fibula complex fractures. She is on bed rest. All her vital signs are within normal parameters, although her pulse rate is high at 90 beats per minute. She tells you she is in pain and has not had a cigarette 'for ages' and that she is 'gasping for a ciggie'. You are very busy seeing to another patient when Sarah shouts out that she needs the commode urgently. You tell her you are too busy. When you finish what you are doing you go to Sarah and see that she has 'wet herself'. You tut at her and say that she will have to wait to be cleaned up. Sarah starts to cry.

Look at the case study above. What are Sarah's nursing care needs? How you would address them? What aspects were left wanting in the scenario outlined in the case study? Do you think that Sarah was treated with care and compassion?

Activity 1.2

List what you think might be the four most frequent complaints received by The Patients Association from patients about their health care.

It is true to say that reports of poor care seem to dominate the media at present, and in many cases care standards are not being met. However, it is also true that the overwhelming majority of staff working in the care system are skilled and hard-working. But we do need to learn from our mistakes in order to raise standards.

TEST YOUR KNOWLEDGE

1   Name the six components of the culture of compassionate care.

KEY POINTS

- Care and compassion in nursing.
- The culture of compassionate care.
- The principles of nursing practice.

Bibliography

Department of Health and NHS Commissioning Board (2012) *Developing the Culture of Compassionate Care: Creating a New Vision for Nurses, Midwives and Care-givers*. Consultation/discussion paper. Department of Health, London.

Dreaper, J. (2012) *Campaign to Show 'Skill and Compassion' of Nurses*. BBC News, Health, 17 September. wwwnews.live.bbc.co.uk/news/health-19602792.

Nursing and Midwifery Council (2010) Code of Conduct. NMC. London. www.nmc-uk.org

Patients Association, The (2011) *We've Been Listening, Have You Been Learning?* The Patients Association, Harrow.

Royal College of Nursing (2012) *This is Nursing*. http://thisisnursing.rcn.org.uk/.

Royal College of Nursing (2010) *Principles of Nursing Practice*. www.rcn.org.uk/nursingprinciples.

Chapter 2

. . . .

BASIC INFECTION CONTROL AND ASEPTIC TECHNIQUE

Care Skills for Nurses, First Edition. Claire Boyd
© 2014 John Wiley & Sons, Ltd. Published 2014 by John Wiley & Sons, Ltd.

LEARNING OUTCOMES

By the end of this chapter you will have an understanding of basic infection control procedures and the practice of performing aseptic technique.

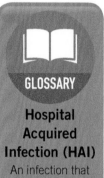

GLOSSARY

Hospital Acquired Infection (HAI)

An infection that a patient did not have prior to being admitted to hospital, but which was contracted in hospital, e.g. MRSA (see Table 2.1).

Adhering to good practice in infection-control principles is a vital and integral part when undertaking any clinical skill in the healthcare environment. It has been estimated that approximately 800 NHS patients contract a hospital-acquired infection every single day while in the care of NHS. Patients also bring with them their own infections when coming into hospital from the community. Estimates are that approximately 5000 patients *die*, per annum, as a direct result of contracting one of these infections. Neonates, the elderly and immunocompromised patients are most at risk because their immune systems cannot fight infections as effectively as others.

As well as the human cost, there are also financial implications for poor hygiene in hosptial. Treatment costs amount to over £1 billion each year, which affects us all as taxpayers.

In the healthcare setting there are micro-organisms all around us that cannot be seen with the naked eye, but which are carried about on bits of dust, fluff, shed skin cells and anything else they can latch on to. Two of the main micro-organism groups are:

- **viruses**, which are smaller than bacteria, e.g. norovirus, which is also known as 'winter vomiting virus' or 'Norwalk virus';
- **bacteria**, which include the 'good bacteria' found on the skin and in the digestive tract, and the 'bad bacteria' such as those responsible for causing Legionnaire's disease, pimples and boils.

VIRUSES

Viruses can be spread; that is why we need to stay off work for 48 hours following an illness, allowing the virus to pass through our system and to 'burn out'. This means 48 hours after the last vomiting or faecal episode. This type of illness is often referred to as D&V, or diarrhoea and vomiting. Viruses can be spread by droplets when someone sneezes or even by indirect spread, such as being picked up from a hard surface by the hands. This is also known as transient spread. Viruses such as the swine flu virus can remain 'live' for 24 hours on hard surfaces and for 20 minutes on soft surfaces, with an incubation period of 2–5 days.

BACTERIA

Resident Bacteria can be friendly – known as resident – and live on or in the body, such as on the skin or in the digestive tract. They are not a problem as long as they remain in the place they should be, such as in the gut or on the skin. An example of this is *Staphylococcus epidermidis*.
Transient This is when bacteria are picked up inadvertently by the hands from surfaces, such as door handles, and enter the body through the eyes or mouth when wiping our eyes or putting our hands to our mouth. There are many different strains of harmful bacteria, such as *Legionella pneumophila*, which causes Legionnaire's disease, and which may be present in a water supply, in pipes, taps or shower heads.

Let's look at some more of these micro-organisms, which you may have heard of in the healthcare environment (see Table 2.1).

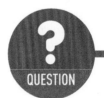

QUESTION

Question 2.1 How do you think the micro-organisms listed in Table 2.1 are spread from person to person?

The spread of infection is usually referred to as the 'chain of infection' (Figure 2.1). A break in the chain will prevent the spread of infection.

Table 2.1 Bacterial infections

Bacterium	Information
Escherichia coli, known as *E. coli*	Friendly bacteria, providing body with many vitamins, such as vitamin K. But strain 0157 is potentially fatal. Its name is Latin for 'of the colon'; it lives in the lower intestines of mammals (gut flora), such as humans and cattle, and can be passed on by eating infected food and liquid. This risk can be minimised by good food-handling practices, ensuring that meat is properly cooked and keeping raw and cooked meats apart.
Clostridium difficile, known as C. diff	Normally found in the digestive tract where the good bacteria keep it under control. But when a patient is receiving antibiotic therapy, or is immunocompromised, elderly or ill, levels of good bacteria are reduced and it becomes possible for C. diff to overpopulate the intestine or colon. It is spread via the faecal/oral route. Yuk! Also, the spores are airborne. C. diff is very 'sticky' and adheres to everything. Ingesting probiotic yoghurt drinks can help the good bacteria to grow back to normal levels, keeping the C. diff under control.
Meticillin-resistant *Staphylococcus aureus*, known as MRSA (note that meticillin was previously known as methicillin)	This bacterium is commonly found on skin and/or in the noses of healthy people: if healthy, colonisation does not cause problems. When MRSA enters the body (e.g. through breaks in the skin) it may cause delayed wound healing. If it enters the lungs it can cause pneumonia. Unfortunately, most strains of *S. aureus* are now resistant to penicillin. Creams, shampoos and mouth antibiotics (nystatin) can be used to get rid of the infection.
MRSA USA 300	This is one of the new boys on the block. It may present as an abscess or boil on the skin, looking like a spider bite. This is a community-acquired infection (CAI) as opposed to a hospital-acquired infection (HAI). It was first found in 2000 in the USA and causes skin and soft tissue damage, pneumonia and/or necrotising fasciitis. It is unusual in that it predominately affects young, fit and healthy people and has been found, and is mainly transmitted, at sports centres, gyms, swimming pools and spas.

Bacterium	Information
Staphylococcus aureus, known as PVL	This is another form of MRSA from the *Staphylococcus* family; many people carry *Staphylococcus* bacteria in their throats. Panton–Valentine leukocidin, or PVL, MRSA strains also affect young, healthy people and destroy white blood cells, which normally fight off infections. If PVL infections spreads to the lungs they may cause fatal pneumonia and even blood poisoning.
Stenotrophomonas maltophilia, known as Steno	One third of all steno cases are fatal. It is found on shower heads, taps and ventilation tubing (in intensive care units) and catheter tubing. A very rare but nasty bacterium.
New Delhi metallo-β-lactamase 1, known as NDM-1	This was first located in New Delhi and brought back to the UK by patients going abroad for their medical treatment. Infections range from mild to severe and some have been fatal. Two types of bacterium have been found to carry this new form of the NDM-1 enzyme, which is resistant to the antibiotic carbapenem: the gut bacterium *E. coli* and one that can invade the lungs, called *Klebsiella pneumoniae*. Both can lead to urinary tract infections and blood poisoning.

- An infectious agent
- A reservoir
- Portal of exit
- Means of transmission
- Portal of entry
- Person at risk

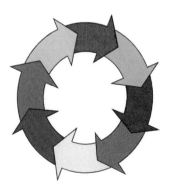

Figure 2.1 The chain of infection. Permission to reproduce this image is granted by North Bristol NHS Trust and University Hospitals Bristol NHS Foundation Trust.

Bacteria love warm, moist areas because they facilitate multiplication, so it is very important to wash and dry the hands after removing gloves, if worn, as the hands may be damp and sweaty. It is also important to keep all equipment, such as wash bowls, dry. The exception to this rule is spacers, the plastic devices that get attached to inhalers. Spacers should be cleaned with soap and water and left to drip dry.

HAND WASHING

Washing the hands with liquid soap is the gold standard of hand hygiene. Alcohol hand gels and antimicrobial detergents may also be used for hand cleaning. Using soap bars in communal areas transfers bugs from person to person, as dead skin cells that have been sloughed off while washing get left on the soap. A liquid soap should be used.

Hands should be **wet** before applying the liquid soap and then rubbed vigorously to remove any contaminants and the dead skin cells. The tap should be run continuously during the hand-washing process. MRSA can survive on skin cells for anything up to 3 hours, so there is little point in performing hand hygiene if you don't remove the bugs! Hands should then be dried well, and in the work environment this should be with single-use towels. What you use at home is a different matter entirely. As our hands are our 'work tools' they should be kept well moisturised and supple to prevent cracks, through which micro-organisms can enter.

Hand Hygiene

Many of us think that we clean our hands thoroughly, when in actual fact we usually miss whole areas of the hand. The dark areas in Figure 2.2 show the areas that are most frequently missed, with the lighter areas showing where people have better success rates, when audits have been performed. So, the dark areas can potentially harbour all sorts of micro-organisms that can be passed on by transfer.

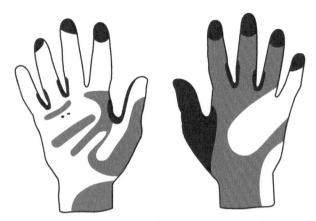

Figure 2.2 Areas of the hands that get missed during hand washing: darker areas are the most frequently missed. Permission to reproduce this image is granted by North Bristol NHS Trust and University Hospitals Bristol NHS Foundation Trust.

As part of infection-control measures some NHS trusts also ask staff to remove engraved wedding bands, as the engravings may be contaminated with germs, especially those with 'stones' (gems, etc.). Only plain wedding bands are permitted, and certainly no engagement rings or other jewellery, which as well as harbouring germs may cut and mark our patient. Nail varnish and 'gel' false nails also attract micro-organisms (especially the 'sticky' C. diff) and staff are therefore not permitted to wear them.

This policy is called **naked to the elbow**, meaning tips of the fingers up to the elbow, not toes up to the elbow: that would be a step too far, if not a little chilly during winter months! Medics going into clinical areas are also required to roll up their sleeves in line with this principle, and in some areas even have to remove their ties in case they are contaminated with micro-organisms. 'White coats' are now seldom seen.

Hand-Washing Procedure

Hand washing – when performed correctly – is universally considered to be the most effective infection-control measure. To make sure that every part of the hand has been cleaned a technique known as the six-point hand-wash technique is used. This technique should also be used when using alcohol gel on the hands.

After wetting the hands and squirting on some liquid soap and working it into a frothy lather, follow these simple steps:

1. rub hands palm to palm,
2. rub right palm over left dorsum and left palm over right dorsum,
3. rub hands palm to palm with the fingers interlaced,
4. rub backs of fingers to opposing palms with fingers interlocked,
5. perform a rotational rubbing movement of the right thumb clasped in the left palm and vice versa,
6. perform a rotational rubbing backwards and forwards movement with clasped fingers of right hand in left palm and vice versa.

Finish with wiping the wrists. Dry the hands thoroughly with a single-use towel.

This whole procedure should take **approximately 15–30 seconds**.

Many healthcare areas now ask staff to prove their competence in regard to effective hand hygiene, assessing staff in their technique (Figure 2.3).

Competence	Achieved		Date	If not competent please write feedback and date for next assessment
	Yes	No		
Correct hand-washing technique				
Correct application of hand gel				

Figure 2.3 Evidence of hand-hygiene practice. Permission to reproduce this image in part is granted by North Bristol NHS Trust and University Hospitals Bristol NHS Foundation Trust.

When to Wash the Hands

Hands should always be washed prior to undertaking any **aseptic technique**, such as performing a urinary catheterisation.

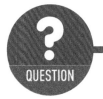

QUESTION

Question 2.2 When else should you wash your hands? List 10 examples, if you can.

The times to wash the hands have been broken down and are often referred to as the World Health Organization's 'Five moments for hand hygiene':

1   before patient contact,
2   before an aseptic task,
3   after body-fluid exposure risk,
4   after patient contact,
5   after contact with patient surroundings.

Alcohol Gel

Alcohol gel is good to use during clinical procedures, when we can't leave our patient to go to a sink and wash our hands. In such cases a container of alcohol gel on the bottom shelf of the trolley means that the patient doesn't need to be left alone for the nurse to maintain hand hygiene. In community settings it is also very useful to use alcohol gel in a service user's home, if at any time a clean sink is not accessible to wash the hand with soap and water.

NOTE: alcohol gel **must not be used** where there are outbreaks of C. diff and norovirus as only soap and water is effective against these micro-organisms.

Wearing Gloves

Gloves used in health care tend to be made of latex, nitrile (latex-free) or vinyl. They can be sterile or 'socially clean'.

It is socially clean gloves we use for most day-to-day tasks, with sterile gloves being used for all aseptic techniques. Most gloves are a uniform shape, with no specific right- or left-hand glove, although some are presented in this form.

Fill a latex glove with water, tie the end and place it in a tray. The next day you will find a deflated glove sitting in a large pool of water. This is because the gloves have microscopic holes. Did you wonder why in the When to Wash your Hands section it was stated that you needed to wash your hands **before** putting on the gloves, as well as **after** removing them? This is because, just as the water can transfer out through the latex, so can any bugs on your hands.

Latex gloves must not be used by any individual with a latex allergy, and those allergic to avocados, bananas and kiwi fruit. This is due to the fact that these fruits contain the same protein as the rubber plant, and ingesting these food stuffs can set off a reaction, such as full-blown anaphylaxis. Chapter 8 explains this is fuller detail.

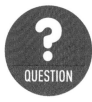

Question 2.3   When would you wear gloves? Give as many examples as you can.

APRONS

Aprons are single-use, which means that they must be removed after the task and a new apron donned for other tasks. Aprons should also be removed appropriately:

* break the ties around the neck and waist,
* pull the apron away from the neck and shoulders, lifting over the head, touching the inside only,
* screw the apron into a ball and dispose.

A clean apron must be worn during each task.

PERSONAL PROTECTIVE EQUIPMENT

When required to wear personal protective equipment – known as PPE – this equipment should be put on and removed in a set sequence. Order of putting on:

1   apron (or gown),
2   mask or respirator,
3   eye protection,
4   gloves.

Order of taking off:

1   gloves,
2   apron (or gown),
3   eye protection,
4   mask or respirator.

UNIFORMS

Staff who wear uniforms should wear a clean one every day, adequately laundering them between uses. Staff should never wear their uniform in public places, such as supermarkets. The public are quite rightly very concerned when they see health carers in public places, being aware that they may be spreading hospital micro-organisms as they lean over the fruit and vegetables while shopping after they have come off duty.

If a uniform must be worn while travelling to and from work then an outer garment should be worn to cover the uniform.

Community staff should always wear suitable outer garments when out and about.

ASEPTIC TECHNIQUE

Many clinical skills, such as wound care and surgical procedures, must be performed in the complete absence of micro-organisms, known as an **aseptic technique**. This is a step above a clean technique. A **clean technique** is

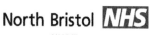

North Bristol **NHS**

NHS Trust

Aseptic and Aseptic Non Touch Technique Competency Framework

This assessment document should be used in conjunction with local clinical guidelines / care bundles.

Name .... Date of formal training or observed assessment ....

Assessors must assess against the following criteria for insertion and ongoing care action competence.

Knowledge

		Competent		Date	Assessor's feedback
		YES	NO		
1	Identify local policy: Infection Control Policy IC01/05/06/09/10				
2	Able to identify the continuing clinical indication for performing the procedure				
3	Can identify Trust Wound Product Formulary or as indicated by Wound Assessment and Management Care Plan or guidelines / care bundle for wound management				

Risk Management

		Competent		Date	Assessor's feedback
		YES	NO		
1	Knowledge of incident reporting policy CG01 (AIMS)				
2	Consent policy CG07 and issues in clinical practice. Able to identify how to proceed if the patient lacks capacity				
3	Identify and discuss the following hazards: • Pain • Potential infection risk • Contamination of specimen samples • Allergies / sensitivities to product used in the procedure & alternative preparations • Needle stick injury				

Procedure

		Competent		Date	Assessor's feedback
		YES	NO		
1	**Staff** • Identify reasons for procedure / frequency				
2	**Patient** • Clinical observations • Providing information related to the intended procedure • Consent • Positioning • Environment • Allergies / sensitivities				

P/ infection control/ DOH/ Aseptic and Aseptic Non Touch Technique competency framework V3
Aug 2011

Figure 2.4 *(continued)*

3	**Equipment cleaning and preparation for the procedure** • Trolley cleaning & preparation • Selects appropriate sterile packs and individual components required to complete the procedure • Able to identify appropriate dressing type and or resource				
4	**Hand hygiene** • Technique prior to procedure				
5	**Personal protective equipment** • Correct use of PPE • Patient barrier drapes (if applicable)				
6	**Site and dressing inspection** • Removal of dressing (if applicable) • Frequency • Site visible / observation				
7	**Skin preparation** • Appropriate skin preparation cleansing prior to procedure (e.g. pre operative / cannulation skin prep -if applicable)				
8	**Procedure** • Aseptic Non Touch Technique • Appropriate wound cleansing procedure (if applicable) • Dressing applied as per guidelines / care bundle				
9	**Disposal** • Clinical waste • Equipment / instruments • Sharps				
10	**Hand hygiene** • Technique during and post procedure				
11	**Documentation** • Aseptic technique intervention documentation				

Evidence of Practice

Date:	Competent		Comments
	YES	NO	

SIGNATURE OF ASSESSOR: ....

PRINT FULL NAME: ....

P/ infection control/ DOH/ Aseptic and Aseptic Non Touch Technique competency framework V3
Aug 2011

Figure 2.4 Aseptic and aseptic non-touch technique competency documentation. Permission to reproduce this image is granted by North Bristol NHS Trust and University Hospitals Bristol NHS Foundation Trust.

when we wash our hands and put on non-sterile gloves. An example of this is when assisting someone in the clinical procedure of clean intermittent catheterisation.

We also need to be aware of the **no-touch technique**: this is when the clean hands must not contaminate any sterile equipment or patients. An example of this technique is when we are performing a urinary catheterisation, wearing clean gloves, and need to pick up the cleaning materials from a laid-out dressing pack to clean the meatus. The gloves are removed before cleaning the hands with alcohol gel, donning sterile gloves and going on to clean the meatus using aseptic technique.

As part of the Department of Health's *Saving Lives* campaign, aiming to reduce infections across the healthcare environment, staff should undergo assessment in order to prove competence in the aseptic and aseptic non-touch techniques. An example of this competency documentation is shown in Figure 2.4.

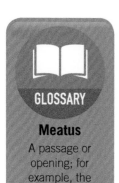

GLOSSARY

Meatus

A passage or opening; for example, the urethral meatus is the external opening of the urethra.

TEST YOUR KNOWLEDGE

1   What are the five moments for hand hygiene?
2   Which areas of the hands are frequently missed during hand washing?
3   Why is it important that wrist and hand jewellery are removed before entering clinical areas?
4   What is the name of the hand-wash technique that uses using soap and water?
5   What is the technique called when using alcohol gel?
6   What is MRSA USA 300?

KEY POINTS

- Bacteria and viruses.
- The chain of infection.
- Hand hygiene.
- Personal protection equipment.
- Aseptic and aseptic non touch technique.

Bibliography

Department of Health (2000) *Saving Lives: a Delivery Programme to Reduce Healthcare Associated Infection including MRSA.* Department of Health, London.

Dougherty, L. and Lister, S. (eds) (2011) *The Royal Marsden Hospital Manual of Clinical Nursing Procedures*, 8th edn. Wiley-Blackwell, Oxford.

National Patient Safety Agency (2008) *Clean Hands Save Lives. Patient Safety Alert*, 2nd edn. National Patient Safety Agency, London.

Taylor, L. (1978) An evaluation of hand washing technique. *Nursing Times* 74(3), 108–110.

World Health Organization (2000) *A Guide to the Implementation of the WHO Multimodal Hand Hygiene Improvement Strategy.* World Health Organization, Geneva.

Website

The BBC Health homepage: www.bbc.co.uk/news/health

Chapter 3

· · · · · · · · · · · · · · · · · · · ·

PERFORMING
PERSONAL CARE

Care Skills for Nurses, First Edition. Claire Boyd
© 2014 John Wiley & Sons, Ltd. Published 2014 by John Wiley & Sons, Ltd.

Performing personal care on patients and service users is done not only for hygiene purposes but also for their psychological well-being. Cleanliness should be seen as a basic human right. Providing personal care is part of the holistic approach to patient care and you may be required to assist the patient in showering, bathing, mouth care, and eye and ear care as well as nail care. Some patients may refer to their daily hygiene care as their 'ablutions' or 'toilet' (sometimes said in a French accent)!

Care that is provided can be very intimate in nature, so you may need to consider chaperoning while you perform this skill, if appropriate. As in all nursing activities self-care should always be promoted whenever the patient is able, but if a person is so incapacitated then we are required to undertake their personal care for them, such as performing a bed bath. While performing this type of care we can assess skin integrity and changes in our patient's mood and pain levels. Sometimes care of this nature is the only personal contact that an individual receives, so it is considered our honour to care for them in this very intimate aspect of nursing.

Before providing personal care, as with all clinical skills, consent must be obtained prior to commencing the procedure. After the procedure all clinical skills performed in relation to the patient's personal care must be documented.

SKIN CARE

The skin is a truly wonderful organ and I have found no better quote, although somewhat dated, than the following:

There is no magician's mantle to compare with the skin in its diverse roles of waterproof, overcoat, sunshade, suit of armour and refrigerator, sensitive to the touch of a feather, to temperature and to pain, withstanding the wear and tear of three score years and ten and executing its own running repairs.

Lockhart et al. (1974)

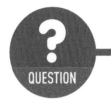

Question 3.1 Before you look at Table 3.1, try to list as many of the skin's main functions as you can.

QUESTION

The skin's main functions are detailed in Table 3.1 (other aspects of the skin's structure and function are described in Chapters 5 and 12).

Table 3.1 Functions of the skin

Skin function	Information
Heat regulation	The skin helps with the regulation of body temperature: it does this by the blood vessels expanding (vasodilatation) when it is hot. The capillaries dilate so that more blood reaches the surface of the skin, allowing heat to escape the body. The body's metabolic rate also increases and the body sweats, allowing cooling by evaporation of moisture from the skin. To raise body temperature the capillaries contrict (vasoconstriction), thus diverting blood from the skin, the sweat pores close and blood moves to organs to ensure they are maintained. We also shiver, which produces warmth in our muscles and helps us to warm up.
Protection	The skin is one of the main protective organs of the body. It protects the deeper and more delicate structures, and acts as the main barrier against the invasion of microbes and other harmful agents. Due to the presence of the sensory nerve endings in the skin, the body reacts by reflex action to unpleasant or painful stimuli, protecting it from further injury. The skin stores water and fat and prevents water loss.

(continued)

Table 3.1 *(Continued)*

Skin function	Information
Absorption	The skin allows fine particles to be admitted and this is called absorption. Some drugs such as hormone-replacement therapy (for menopausal women) can be given as either skin patches or in cream form, and drugs such as nicotine may be applied via patches to smoking cessation. Essential oils in aromatherapy are absorbed by the skin because the molecules are so small, but it must be remembered these oils can be toxic so must be used with care. Other substances that are toxic to the body and composed of small molecules can also enter the skin. One example is mercury, so take care if you break an old-fashioned thermometer not to touch the silver fluid.
Excretion	The body uses the skin as an excretory organ to rid itself of toxins in the fastest possible way. This is via pores in the form of sweat or perhaps as spots.
Secretion	The skin's secretory functions are a protection mechanism: sebaceous glands secrete sebum which protects the skin against fungal and bacterial infection. Sweat glands expel sweat, playing a key role in thermoregulation by initiating evaporative cooling.
Vitamin D formation	Vitamin D_3 is formed from the fatty substance 7-dehydrocholesterol plus ultraviolet light from the sun's rays. This is used together with calcium and phosphorous in the formation and maintenance of strong bones. Any excess vitamin is not wasted as it is stored in the liver for use when needed.
Sensation	The skin contains sensory nerves which cause a reflex action, sending messages to the hypothalamus when sensing heat, cold, pressure and pain. This helps to prevent injury, e.g. retracting a hand from a hot iron to prevent burning and tissue damage. The lips and the fingertips have a higher concentration of sensory receptors, which is why we enjoy kissing!

THE SKIN AND THE AGEING PROCESS

When a person is in their early 20s the skin should be at its best. In the late 20s and early 30s fine lines appear on the skin's surface, especially around the eyes where the skin is thinner. After 40 years, hormone activity in the body slows down so the sebaceous glands produce less sebum and the skin becomes increasingly drier. Lines and wrinkles appear on the surface. Wrinkling is due to changes in the collagen and elastin fibres of the connective tissue. The collagen fibres in the dermis begin to decrease in number, stiffen and break apart. The elastin fibres lose some of their elasticity and break down, so that when the skin is stretched it does not immediately return to its original state when the stretching stops. In people who are regularly exposed to ultraviolet light or who smoke, the loss of elasticity of the skin is greatly accelerated. Repeated facial expressions cause 'crow's feet' to form at the side of the eyes.

As a person reaches their late 50s brown patches of discoloured skin, called lentigines ('liver spots'), may appear on the back of hands and temple areas because of an increase in the size of some melanocytes. The blood flow to the liver spots is reduced, and the rate of mitosis in the basal layer slows down. The horny layer is therefore thinner, making the skin more fragile. Dilated capillaries appear, especially on the cheeks and nose. Sebaceous glands decrease in size, which leads to dry and cracked skin. The sweat glands are less active and loss of subcutaneous fat often occurs (causing 'tissue-paper' skin).

Hair growth slows down and a decrease in the number of functioning melanocytes results in grey hairs. The skin of elderly people heals poorly and becomes susceptible to infection.

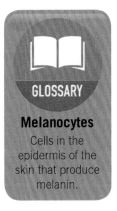

GLOSSARY

Melanocytes

Cells in the epidermis of the skin that produce melanin.

CARING FOR BABIES AND INFANTS SKIN

Babies have very delicate skin which can be sensitive to their new environment, away from the mother's moist, temperature-controlled womb. This makes little ones prone to skin irritation and dryness. As soon as a baby has soiled their nappy, the nappy should be changed. Otherwise the faeces and urine can break down the skin, causing 'nappy rash'. Babies should be bathed regularly and lotion applied to their skin to prevent the skin from getting too dry.

Fragrance-free lotions are best for a baby's sensitive skin because the fragrances may irritate the skin.

Even as the infant grows, fragrance-free products should be used so as not to irritate the skin, using gentle soaps to wash the child's body. Rub soap into a sponge and work from the head down, and gently working between the skin folds, checking the thighs, bottom and genitals for signs of nappy rash if the infant is still wearing nappies.

Encourage the child to take part in bathing, making it a fun experience and getting the child involved. Teaching children the importance of good hand hygiene can never be started at too early an age.

BED BATHING

If, for whatever reason, a patient is unable to wash in the bathroom or take a shower themselves we may need to perform a bed bath. Not performing good daily skin hygiene – washing – will make a patient more prone to developing an infection. We must always involve the patient in their plan of care, as we all have our own preferences for toiletries, etc. Other considerations must include a patient's cultural or religious beliefs. The patient must be given privacy and treated with dignity, and the environment must be warm and draft-free.

Bed bathing is the ideal opportunity to conduct a thorough inspection of the skin, observing for pressure ulcers, marks, breaks in the skin, bruising, etc. Delicate skin will require extra care with washing and patting the skin dry.

The Bed Bath Procedure

Equipment
Clean nightwear or clothes
Apron
Gloves
Clinical waste bag
Shaving equipment
Manual handling equipment, e.g. glide sheet

Equipment
Clean bed linen
Laundry skip
Bowl of water, hand hot
Soap and disposable wash cloths
Patient's choice of toiletries
Two or three towels

1   Gain consent from the patient and then explain the procedure.

2   Ensure the area is warm and that privacy is maintained.

3   Prepare all equipment.

4   Wash hands and put on an apron.

5   Offer the patient a bed pan prior to the procedure.

6   Ask the patient to test the water temperature.

7   Cover the patient with a towel and, after asking if they wish to have soap on their face, wash the patient's face. Rinse with water and dry. The patient may be able to assist with this part of the procedure.

8   Remove the patient's upper garments and place a towel under one arm and wash this upper limb, starting with the arm furthest away from you. Cover the arm not being washed with a towel. If two nurses are present for this procedure the second nurse can dry the first arm while the first nurse washes the other one.

9   Apply any toiletries that have been requested, e.g. deodorant, and apply clean clothing.

10   Repeat the procedure for the lower limbs. Put on gloves.

11   Roll the patient on to their side using the correct manual handling equipment. Place a towel lengthwise as far under the patient's body as possible and wash and dry the patient's back and buttocks. Check the skin integrity at all times.

12   Change the water at this point, or sooner if it is becoming dirty and cold. Wash the genitalia using a different wash cloth.

13   Replace clothing or nightwear. Put compression stockings on the patient, if required.

14   Roll the patient again and insert clean bed linen underneath their body, pulling out the dirty bed sheets.

15   Cover the patient with top bedding.

16   Reposition the patient and make them comfortable.

17   Perform mouth care.

18   Shave the patient, if required.

19   Brush the patient's hair.

20   Wash and dispose of equipment and dirty bedding, wash and dry the bowl and put the patient's belongings in their locker.

21   Document all care that has been provided.

NOTE: if the patient wears glasses or contact lenses you will need to clean these, before assisting the patient to replace them, if required. If the patient has an artificial eye care will be required to keep it clean: specialist advice should be sought for this care.

COMPRESSION STOCKINGS

After a bed bath compression stockings may need to be applied. Compression stockings are worn to help to maintain circulation and reduce the risk of blood clots forming in the veins of the legs (known as deep-vein thrombosis or DVT). Compression stockings are also called thrombo-embolic deterrent stockings, or TEDS.

Compression stockings are constructed from elastic fibres or rubber. These fibres help to compress the limb, decreasing the diameter of the veins, and are used to support the venous and lymphatic systems of the leg. Depending on the amount of compression applied, some stockings or socks can be brought over the counter in a pharmacy (e.g. 'flight socks'). Others will need to be prescribed.

Stockings may be applied, if clinically warranted, during:

- prolonged bed rest (reduced mobility),
- surgery: especially if lasting for more than 30 minutes,
- surgery involving leg joints or pelvis,

- when taking certain medicines (e.g. contraceptive pill, hormone-replacement therapy),
- pregnancy and childbirth.

Other indications for use include:

- tired, aching legs,
- varicose veins,
- venous insufficiency,
- oedema (swelling in leg),
- lymphoedema,
- burn scarring,
- long-haul aeroplane journeys.

Compression stockings are available in a wide range of colours and sizes. They also come in three styles.

QUESTION

Question 3.2 What do you think are the three styles of compression stockings?

The different compression stocking styles will require different fitting instructions. Thigh-high stockings tend to be fitted according to the manufacturer's instructions by measuring:

a   widest part of the thigh,
b   widest part of the calf,
c   just above the malleolus (ankle bone),
d   from back of heel to the longest toe.

Procedure for Applying Compression Stockings

1   Insert your hand into the stocking as far as the heel pocket.
2   Turn the stocking inside out.

3   Carefully slip the service user's foot into the sock and ease the stocking over the heel. Check that the heel fits into the heel pocket.

4   Bring the rest of the stocking over the heel, up around the ankle and calf. Don't pull the stocking: gently massage it upwards using the palm of your hands.

MOUTH CARE

Good oral hygiene should be performed on patients at least on a daily basis, as poor hygiene in the mouth can be associated with painful, unpleasant diseases such as gingivitis and halitosis. Poor oral hygiene can also be linked to infections and pneumonia.

Oral assessment includes a visual examination of the oral cavity and teeth. The oral mucosa and tongue should be pink and moist, with smooth moist lips and clean teeth (or well-fitted dentures if they are worn). Oral infections can present as sore, reddened areas. Fungal infections to the mucosa and tongue may present with a creamy, white coating, and both these conditions must be acted on immediately by securing medical intervention.

The Mouth Care Procedure

Equipment
Clean tray
Mouth wash
Plastic disposable cup
Denture pot (if required)
Foam mouth-care sticks
Tissues
Wooden spatula
Toothbrush
Gloves
Apron
Clinical waste bag

1. Explain the procedure to the patient.
2. Wash hands and put on gloves (non-latex).
3. If the patient has dentures, remove them and place in a denture pot.
4. Put a small amount of toothpaste on a toothbrush or foam stick and gently brush the patient's teeth, gums and tongue (both inner and outer aspects of the teeth).
5. Give the patient a cup of water or mouthwash for them to rinse out their mouth, or perform this for the patient by wetting a foam stick and rotating it around the mouth.
6. If the lips are dry, apply a lubricant.
7. If the patient wears dentures, clean them with a toothbrush, and rinse and replace them in the patient's mouth.
8. Dispose of used equipment.
9. Clean the toothbrush and leave to dry.
10. Wash hands.

EAR, EYE AND NOSE CARE

Part of a patient's personal care includes care of the ears, eyes and nose. Build up of wax in the ear canals can result in impairment of hearing and should be reported.

Patients with nasogastric tubes or those having oxygen therapy administered should have regular reviews to avoid excessive drying and/or excoriation of the nasal passages.

NAIL CARE

Fingernails should be trimmed correctly to avoid pain and infection. Patients who need their toenails to be trimmed should be referred to the chiropodist. In particular, patients with diabetes should only have their toenails trimmed by a chiropodist due to the potential risk of skin breakdown.

TEST YOUR KNOWLEDGE

1   Name six of the main functions of the skin.
2   What are the three styles of compression stocking?
3   A bed bath is an ideal time to conduct which sorts of patient assessment?
4   Patients with diabetes should only have their nails cut by which of the following: (a) qualified nurse/midwife; (b) a doctor; (c) a chiropodist; (d) anyone can cut the nails if they require trimming.

KEY POINTS

- Skin care.
- The skin and the ageing process.
- Caring for babies and infants skin.
- Bed bathing.
- Compression stockings.
- Mouth care.
- Ear, eye and nose care.
- Nail care.

Bibliography

Dawney, L. and Lloyd, H. (2008) Bed bathing patients in hospital. Clinical Skills. *Nursing Standard* 22, 34–40.

Dougherty, L. and Lister, S. (eds) (2011) *The Royal Marsden Hospital Manual of Clinical Nursing Procedures*, 8th edn. Wiley-Blackwell, Oxford.

Lockhart, R.D., Hamilton, G.F. and Fyfe, F.W. (1974) *Anatomy of the Human Body*. Faber and Faber, London.

Pegram, A., Bloomfield, J. and Jones, A. (2007). Clinical skills bed bathing and personal hygiene needs of patients. *British Journal of Nursing* 16(6), 356–358.

Chapter 4
CONTINENCE CARE

Care Skills for Nurses, First Edition. Claire Boyd
© 2014 John Wiley & Sons, Ltd. Published 2014 by John Wiley & Sons, Ltd.

LEARNING OUTCOMES

By the end of this chapter you will have an understanding of the theory and practice of performing the clinical skill of continence care.

One thing we can all be sure about is that at some point(s) during the day we will all need to void bodily waste by the acts of urination (micturition) or elimination of faeces (or stools); or, to put it in its simplest form, to 'wee and poo'.

URINE

Urine is secreted into the bladder throughout the day but production slows down during sleep. Therefore the first void after waking is usually more concentrated and darker in colour. Urine should be what is described as a 'straw-coloured' but does vary, sometimes being closer to amber in colour.

Urine can also take on other colours due to factors such as disease, medications, fluid intake, infection, trauma or diet.

Activity 4.1

ACTIVITY

Figure 4.1 shows the colour of four samples of urine that you may see in catheter-drainage bags. What do you think has caused the colouration of the urine in each case?

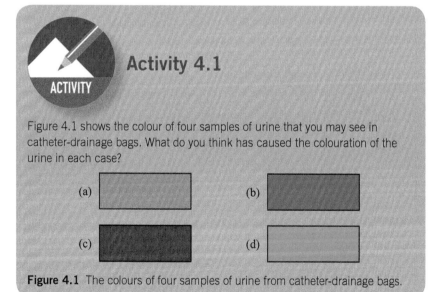

(a)   (b)   (c)   (d)

Figure 4.1 The colours of four samples of urine from catheter-drainage bags.

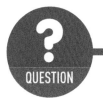

Question 4.1 What is urine comprised of? Should protein be present in urine?

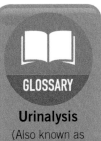

GLOSSARY

Urinalysis

(Also known as a 'urine dipstick' test) A test to establish the pH of urine and what substances or cell types are present, such as protein, glucose, ketones, blood, leucocytes and nitrites.

The specific gravity of urine is between 1.015 and 1.025 – this means the relative **density** – and is acidic in nature with a pH of about 6 (anything from 4.5 to 8). Drinking more results in a higher urine output and drinking less leads to a decreased urine output. Fresh urine should only have a very slight smell but when exposed to air it starts to decomposes and begins to smell very strongly of ammonia.

Micturition, or the discharge of urine, usually occurs around five to ten times per day in the average person, who produces about 1–1.5 litres each day. However, I have yet to meet this 'average' person!

When we feel the desire to void most of us can suppress it for a considerable period of time, until there is a suitable time and place.

Urinary Incontinence

Incontinence is the *involuntary* passing of urine in *inappropriate* places at *inappropriate* times. According to the Department of Health, urinary incontinence is:

> The most commonly seen problem facing carers, both in hospital and in the community, yet it is probably the most misunderstood and therefore mismanaged condition.

> Department of Health (2000)

Many individuals do not seek help with their urinary incontinence as they often feel too embarrassed about their condition. However, with understanding and careful management many patients can achieve continence or partial continence. Urinary incontinence is known as **enuresis**.

Facts and Figures

- The average Primary Care Trust (when they still existed) had approximately 5600 people with urinary incontinence and 900 people with faecal incontinence.
- One person in six over the age of 40 years is incontinent 'several times a month'.
- Incontinence is very common in women after childbirth and during the menopause.
- It is very common in men in later life (especially those with prostate conditions).

Source: www.bladderandbowelfoundation.org.

Babies and Children

Newborn babies excrete urine from the urinary bladder after birth as a reflex when the bladder is full. It is an involuntary response. Voluntary control is usually achieved by the age of 3 years. If healthy children continue to wet themselves after the age of 5, or regress to this behaviour pattern after a period of dryness, they are described as experiencing urinary incontinence.

Night-time bed wetting is known as nocturnal enuresis, and is usually treated with a variety of techniques, one of which is based on the conditioning principle. Here, the child is woken during the night and taken to the toilet.

Types and Causes of Urinary Incontinence

When caring for people with urinary incontinence it is very important that we know what type of urinary incontinence the individual is experiencing so that we can provide the correct care. The term **neurogenic bladder** is used when there is interference with the nerve supply to the bladder, which can result in various forms of incontinence. Six types of urinary incontinence are presented in Table 4.1.

Table 4.1 Types of urinary incontinence

Type of urinary incontinence	Presentation	Possible causes
1 Stress incontinence	Slight leakage of urine during any physical activity (sneezing, coughing, jogging, laughing) due to a rise in abdominal pressure	Pregnancy, childbirth, oestrogen withdrawal in menopause, obesity, pelvic-floor weakness, prostatic surgery
2 Urgency/urge incontinence	Individual experiences an involuntary loss of urine, accompanied by a strong desire to void	Detrusor muscle instability, central nervous system problems e.g. stroke (cerebrovascular accident), Parkinson's disease, multiple sclerosis, bladder or Brain tumour, urinary tract infection, long-term indwelling catheter
3 Overflow incontinence	Involuntary, unpredictable loss of urine in the presence of a residual amount of urine in the bladder. Causes a stream of urine, leading to constant dampness, or may need to strain to void	Sensory peripheral neuropathy (diabetic), spina bifida, Parkinson's disease, faecal impaction, urethral strictures, lower sacral cord injury, some anti-depressants
4 Reflex incontinence	Involuntary loss of urine when certain bladder volume is reached	Cerebrovascular accident, dementia, confusion, spinal injury above the level of S2, spina bifida
5 Environmental/ locomotor incontinence	Leakage of urine due to inability to toilet themselves	Cognitive impairment, confusion, physical disabilities
6 Functional incontinence	Leakage of urine due to functional problems	Cognitive impairment, poor manual dexterity, sensory deficits, depression, alcoholism, reduction in mobility, sedatives, diuretics

Promoting Continence

The following are some of the areas which may need to be addressed when an individual is experiencing urinary incontinence:

- **pelvic-floor exercises:** to strengthen this muscle set,
- **bladder retraining:** to establish a regular pattern; keeping a bladder diary,
- **adequate toileting:** the individual may require assistance to toilet and we may consider aids, such as commodes, bedpans and urinals, and always remember to put them within easy reach,
- **treat underlying disorders:** avoid constipation and assess for urinary tract infections by obtaining a urine sample and performing an urinalysis,
- **adequate fluid intake:** the individual is encouraged to drink adequate fluids and to review fluid types, such as bladder irritants such as coffee and cola (caffeine-based beverages),
- **drug therapy:** a GP may review present medications, such as sedatives,
- **surgery:** a GP may refer the person to a continence advisor or urologist,
- **improve environment:** the patient may find it difficult to mobilise to an upstairs toilet. We would need to conduct an assessment to find other factors that may be contributing to the incontinence, e.g. eyesight tests,
- **containment:** e.g. pads/appliances,
- **urinary drainage:** the individual may require urinary catheterisation, either intermittent or indwelling.

We must always report any concerns we have with service users, patients or any individual in our care to a nurse in charge, GP or member of the multidisciplinary team caring for the individual.

There are two main types of incontinence pad:

1. shaped product used in conjunction with a fitting product, e.g. net pants,
2. all-in-one pad (see Figure 4.2).

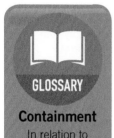

GLOSSARY

Containment

In relation to incontinence, this is when an individual may be required to wear incontinence pads in the short or long term. These pads should never be stored in the bathroom, or any other warm, moist area, as they contain a silicone layer which expands when moist. Incorrect storage will render these pads less effective.

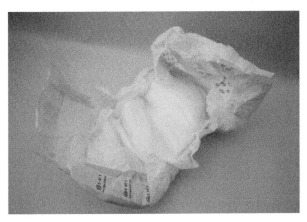

Figure 4.2 Incontinence pad.

The correct fitting of these pads is very important, and these general rules apply:

- do not touch the inside of the pad,
- the pad should fit neatly into the individual's groin,
- the back of the pad should be turned away from the body and groin,
- apply the pad from the front to back and always remove the pad from behind,
- do not use any talcum powder or oil-based barrier creams (which tend to block the pad's top dry layer),
- if an individual's skin is not marked or red, do not apply cream,
- the pad should be changed every 3–4 hours during the day and evening,
- the pad can be used for up to 8 hours during the night to promote adequate sleep patterns,
- do not store pads in a bathroom (damp environment), but in a dry, warm surroundings.

FLUIDS

Encouraging a patient to drink more fluids is often called 'pushing fluids' in health care. We would also encourage drinking more caffeine-free drinks, and also the consumption of foods with a high water content, such as soup, ice cream, etc. However, if an individual loves their cups of tea, and this is the only drink they will take, then we need to go with this, as it is individual choice. Remember: care and compassion.

FAECES

Faecal matter is composed of:

- 75% water,
- 25% solid matter, comprising quantities of dead bacteria, fatty acids, inorganic matter, proteins and undigested dietary fibre.

Faecal matter in the adult is normally brown in colour, soft and cylindrical. Faeces have an odour due to the bacterial flora in the intestine, which varies according to the bacteria present and the food ingested.

The time it takes for undigested food to travel from the mouth through the alimentary canal and then out of the anus is known as the transit time, which is normally anything from 1 to 3 days in a young healthy adult. Older people may have an increased transit time of anything up to 2 weeks.

Babies and Children

Newborn babies excrete meconium waste matter from their bowels in an involuntary fashion. Meconium is a greenish-black sticky substance which consists of mucus, endothelial cells, amniotic fluid, bile pigments and fats. After a few days the stools become a brownish-green in colour, then yellow.

Breast-fed babies produce a softer, brighter yellow stool than bottle-fed infants, whose stools are paler and more formed. Once the child is weaned and eating a balanced diet the faeces become more like an adult's in composition.

Bowel Assessment

When conducting a full bowel assessment, Horton (2004) suggested that the following components should be identified in order for any care package and treatments to commence. Although this article was produced some time ago it still rings true:

- usual stool consistency,
- usual stool frequency,
- pain associated with bowel motion,
- presence of blood and/or mucus,
- evacuation problems,
- past medical history,
- toilet-access issues,
- diet and fluid intake,
- medication, including over-the-counter medications.

Any changes in the normal bowel pattern could indicate bowel dysfunction.

Many healthcare areas use the Bristol Stool Chart, devised by Lewis and Heaton (1997), to monitor a patient's faeces, with types 3 and 4 being suggested as the 'perfect poo'. Figure 4.3 shows the stool types.

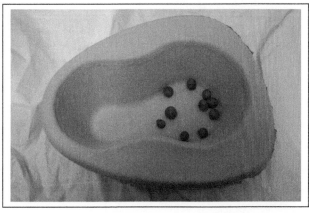

	Type 1 Hard-to-pass hard lumps

Figure 4.3 *(Continued)*

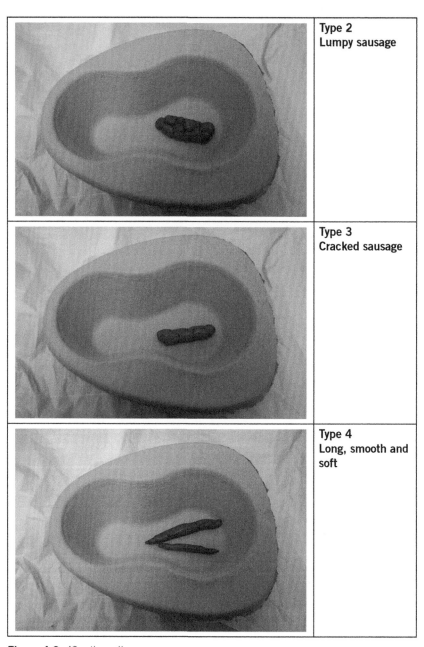

Figure 4.3 *(Continued)*

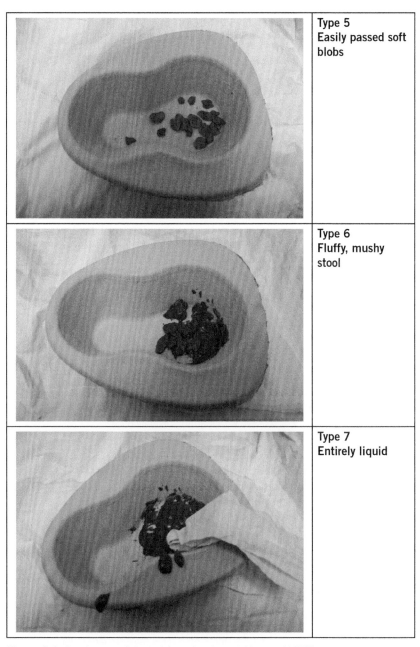

Figure 4.3 Stool types. Adapted from Lewis and Heaton (1997).

Bowel Dysfunction

It has been estimated that 1–10% of adults may experience some form of faecal incontinence, and it is tolerated by carers to a lesser degree than urinary incontinence. For the person involved faecal incontinence is an embarrassing and undignified condition, having a detrimental effect on one's psychological, social and physical well-being.

Causes of Bowel Dysfunction

Groups at high risk of faecal incontinence include (National Institute of Clinical Excellence 2007):

- people with loose stools or diarrhoea from any cause,
- women following child birth (especially following third- or fourth-degree obstetric injury),
- people with neurological or spinal disease (e.g. spina bifida, stroke, multiple sclerosis or spinal cord injury),
- people with severe cognitive impairment,
- people with urinary incontinence,
- people with pelvic organ prolapse and/or rectal prolapse,
- people who have had colonic resection or anal surgery,
- people who have undergone pelvic radiotherapy,
- people with perianal soreness, itching or pain,
- people with learning disabilities.

After a cause has been established, a treatment plan can be initiated. One of the treatment options may include strengthening the pelvic floor muscles. Like all muscles in the body, the more they are used and exercised the stronger and firmer they will become.

Pelvic Floor Exercises

- This pelvic floor exercise can be done sitting down or standing up. Ask the patient to imagine sitting on the toilet passing urine. Now they should imagine stopping the flow of urine, trying to really 'pull' upwards and squeeze and stop it. This may be hard to start with. Some people can manage this upward movement in discrete stages, much like a lift going up past floors in a building! With practise suggest that they try holding for a few seconds and then relaxing and letting go.

- Ask the patient to sit down with the knees slightly apart. Tell them to imagine trying to stop themselves passing wind from the bowel. They should really squeeze and lift the muscle around the back passage. They should feel the skin around the back passage being pulled up and away from the chair and should feel the muscle move, but the buttocks and legs should not move.

These exercises can be done at any time, in any place, and no one need know! Tell the patient not to worry if they cannot feel the muscles very well; over time the pelvic floor will strengthen and tighten and they will gain more control over it.

Another good exercise to strengthen the pelvic floor, as long as the patient does not have back, hip, or knee pain and discomfort, is the pelvic tilt, as follows.

- Tell the patient to stand with feet 30 cm apart and knees slightly bent. Then ask them to rotate their hips in a clockwise circular movement for approximately 10 minutes. They should do this every day.

Other tips to firm up these muscles include avoiding high-impact exercises, which weaken the pelvic floor muscle. In contrast, yoga, pilates, swimming, cycling and belly dancing are considered good exercises for the pelvic floor.

TEST YOUR KNOWLEDGE

1 What is enuresis?
2 What is night-time bed wetting called?
3 Name three types of urinary incontinence.
4 What is the stool of a newborn baby called?
5 What are the questions you should ask the service user or patient when conducting a thorough bowel assessment?
6 Faecal matter is composed of what two things?

KEY POINTS

- The composition of urine and specific gravity.
- Types and causes of urinary incontinence.
- Promoting continence.
- The composition of faeces.
- Causes of bowel dysfunction.

Bibliography

Department of Health (2000) *Good Practice in Continence Services*. Department of Health, London.

Horton, N. (2004) Behavioural and biofeedback therapy for evacuation disorders. In Norton, C. and Chelvanayagam, S. (eds), *Bowel Continence Nursing*. Beaconsfield Publishers, Beaconsfield.

Hung, H.C., Hsiao, S.M., Chih, S.Y. et al. (2010) An alternative intervention for urinary incontinence: retraining diaphragmatic, deep abdominal and pelvic floor muscle co-ordinated function. *Manual Therapy* 15(93), 273–279.

Imamura, M., Abrams, P., Bain, C., Buckley, B., Cardozo, L. et al. (2010) Systematic review and economic modelling of the effectiveness and cost-effectiveness of non-surgical treatments for women with stress urinary incontinence. *Health Technology Assessment* 14(40), whole issue.

Lewis, S.J. and Heaton, K.W. (1997) Stool form scale as a useful guide to intestinal transit time. *Scandinavian Journal of Gastroenterology* 32(9), 920–924.

National Institute of Clinical Excellence (2007) *Faecal Incontinence: the Management of Faecal Incontinence in Adults*. CG49. http://guidance.nice.org.uk/CG49.

Wishin, J., Gallagher, T. and McCann, E. (2008) Emerging options for the management of faecal incontinence in hospitalised patients. *Journal of Wound Ostomy and Continence Nursing* 35(1), 104–110.

Yates, A. (2011) Managing faecal incontinence: a joint approach to guideline development. *Nursing Times* 107, 12.

Website

Bladder and Bowel Foundation (B&BF) homepage: www.bladderandbowelfoundation.org

Chapter 5
. . . .
PRESSURE ULCER CARE

Care Skills for Nurses, First Edition. Claire Boyd
© 2014 John Wiley & Sons, Ltd. Published 2014 by John Wiley & Sons, Ltd.

LEARNING OUTCOMES

By the end of this chapter you will have an understanding of the theory and practice of performing the clinical skill of pressure ulcer care.

'Pressure sore', 'decubitus ulcer' and 'bed sore' are terms that refer to the same problem: skin and/or tissue damage which, if left to progress, may cause an area of skin to become blistered, then ulcerous, causing an open wound. This is the pressure ulcer. Pressure ulcers are defined by the European Pressure Ulcer Advisory Panel (EPUAP) and National Pressure Ulcer Advisory panel (NPUAP) (2009) as:

> A pressure ulcer is localized injury to the skin and/or underlying tissue usually over a bony prominence, as a result of pressure, or pressure in combination with shear.

The term pressure ulcer is generally used rather than 'bed sore', as the latter would indicate that the injury occurred in bed. In fact, any prolonged pressure to particular points on the body – for a variety of different reasons – may cause a pressure ulcer, and not just bed rest.

Once formed, a pressure ulcer can take months to heal, can be quite painful, and in the worst cases can actually become life-threatening.

As part of a drive in the NHS and to reinforce the importance of 'getting it right' the NHS Plan was launched in 2000. The treatment of pressure ulcers costs the NHS in the UK anything between £1.4 and 2.1 billion annually, equating to 4% of total NHS expenditure. Thus the prevention and management of pressure sores has been identified as a key area in healthcare, with the aim of reducing their prevalence.

PRESSURE ULCER ASSESSMENT

Part of the management strategy for pressure ulcers is risk assessment. Risk assessment tools, such as the Waterlow Pressure Ulcer Prevention/Treatment Policy, or

Waterlow risk assessment tool, are used to identify those *at risk* of developing pressure ulcers and are performed on patients when they are first admitted to hospital. Those in the community setting should also have this assessment performed when first coming into contact with health services. As in all health care, good, robust documentation should be implemented.

If these assessments are carried out correctly individuals deemed to be at risk can be prevented from acquiring a pressure ulcer with the help of pressure therapy equipment and strategies used as part of the pressure ulcer prevention strategy. These interventions may include providing equipment such as profiling beds, air flow/foam mattresses and cushions. These are used in conjunction with other nursing interventions, such as turning regimes and regular repositioning and monitoring. Patients assessed as requiring pressure-relieving support will need to continue to receive it 24 hours a day.

A CROSS-SECTION OF THE SKIN

The **epidermis** is the outer coating of the skin and contains no blood vessels or nerve endings. The cells on the surface are continually being rubbed off and replaced by new cells that have arisen from deeper layers. The epidermis has hairs, sweat glands and the ducts of sebaceous glands passing through it.

Underneath the epidermis, the **dermis** is a thicker layer which contains blood vessels, nerve fibres, sweat and sebaceous glands and lymph vessels. It is made up of white fibrous tissue and yellow elastic fibres which give the skin its toughness and elasticity.

The **subcutaneous layer** contains the deep fat cells (areolar and adipose tissue) and has a role in thermoregulation. It also supports the outer layers of the skin (other aspects of the skin's structure and function are described in Chapters 3 and 12).

Pressure ulcers can damage the skin as well as destroy the underlying tissues: the muscle, tendon and bone. However, before the necrotic ulceration stage is reached (see EPUAP grading system section in this chapter), the area of damage may have started as a small area of erythema, which is flushing of the skin caused by the dilation of blood capillaries.

WHAT IS A PRESSURE ULCER?

A pressure ulcer is an area of damage to the skin and underlying tissue that is caused by:

- pressure,
- friction,
- shearing.

Pressure: Weight of the Body Pressing on the Skin

Prolonged pressure from a bed or chair on one side of an area of skin and from bone on the other makes it impossible for the affected area of skin to be properly nourished by tiny blood vessels called capillaries. The area of skin starts to die. The greater the pressure, the more likely it is that damage will occur. This problem is common among people with limited mobility due to disability and/or ill health. Pressure is the single most important factor in the development of pressure ulcers.

Friction: the Result of Two Surfaces Rubbing Together

Friction is another potential cause of pressure ulcers. Movement that causes skin to rub roughly against bedding may damage the capillaries and diminish the blood supply at a particular point. Friction strips the epidermis away, with the resultant exposure of underlying tissue. The effects of friction are exacerbated by moisture.

Shearing: Skin and Muscle Rubbing Together During Movement

Dragging someone across a surface instead of correct manual handling (lifting) can cause damage to the skin by shearing.

HOW TO RECOGNISE A PRESSURE ULCER

A pressure ulcer may be recognised by:

* persistent erythema (redness),
* non-blanching hyperaemia (see the blanch test in the next section),
* blisters,
* skin discolouration,
* localised heat,
* oedema (swelling),
* indurations and a discolouration in those with darkly pigmented skin.

Ideally we need to prevent a pressure ulcer from forming in the first instance, at the very least stopping it from getting worse once it begins to form. It is very important to catch ulcers early. Individuals should be encouraged to inspect their own skin, if possible, as part of a person-centred care approach, and to report any concerns.

TESTING FOR SIGNS OF A PRESSURE ULCER

Patients and clients considered to be at low risk of pressure ulcer development should be checked on a daily basis. Checks should be 4 hourly for those deemed to be at medium risk, and 2 hourly for those considered, via assessment, at high risk.

A pressure ulcer can begin as just a red (on light-skinned individuals) or blue/purple area on a person's skin. If you see this perform the following test, known as blanching hyperaemia, and often referred to as **the blanch test**.

* Press lightly on the reddened/blue/purple area for 10 seconds. If it remains red/blue/purple then this could be an early sign that a pressure ulcer may be developing (known as **non-blanching hyperaemia**).

- If the area of skin goes white/paler (blanches) when pressed and then fades when you stop it may not be a pressure ulcer (known as **blanching hyperaemia**).

Non-blanching hyperaemia indicates that some damage has occurred: **remember, a white mark is not produced**. This is classed as a Grade 1 pressure ulcer according to EPUAP (2003). There is a high risk of further tissue damage occurring unless preventative measures are now taken. It is at this stage that you need to report your concerns to the nurse in charge, or other appropriate person, as tissue death can happen within an hour!

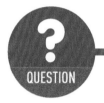

Question 5.1 What do you think are the risk factors for a pressure ulcer? There are 20 to consider.

QUESTION

Other factors

- Clothing and bed linen should be clean and dry.
- Avoid placing heavy objects, such as hot water bottles and heavy bedding, over the body.
- Wound dressings or bandages should not be too tight.
- Correct manual handling techniques should be adhered to at all times.
- Shoes, socks, leg wear (tights, etc.) and compression stockings should not be too tight as to cause problems.

COMMON AREAS FOR PRESSURE AREA FORMATION

Supine position (lying flat on the back of the body):

heels,
sacrum,
elbows,
scapulae,
back of the head.

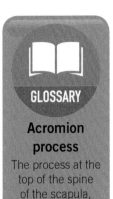

GLOSSARY

Acromion process

The process at the top of the spine of the scapula, part of which articulates with the clavicle.

Prone position (lying flat on the front of the body):

toes,
knees,
genitalia (men),
breasts (women),
acromion process,
cheek and ear.

Lateral position (lying on the side of the body):

malleolus,
medial and lateral condoyle,
greater trochanter,
ribs,
acromion process,
ear.

Sitting position:

back of head,
shoulders,
sacrum,
knee,
feet.

Presentation in infants and children is more likely to occur on the occipital area or ears.

QUESTION

Question 5.2 What are the malleolus and greater tochanter?

CHANGING POSITION

Changing the patient's or client's position is very important for reducing the risk of pressure sores. Also, the the nurse needs to introduce appropriate equipment that is specially designed to spread the weight of the body and to reduce the incidence of pressure ulcer occurrence. Changing the patient's position must take into account their medication condition, as terminal patients and those in high-dependency units require special consideration in pressure ulcer care.

If your patient is confined to a **bed**:

- encourage the patient to change their position approximately every 2 hours, or do this for them,
- avoid allowing your patient to slide down the bed, as this can cause shearing to the skin,
- if assessment has been initiated, use a pressure mattress and cushions and any other appropriate specialised pressure-reliving equipment.

If your patient/clienwt is using a **chair** for long periods, perhaps even sleeping in one, or is in a **wheelchair**:

- ask them to change their position *every hour*, or help them to do so,
- a pressure cushion should *always* be used,
- *do not* use ring- or doughnut-shaped cushions, as these increase pressure to the area of the buttock making contact with the cushion while the main buttock area is in the hole space.

SKIN CARE

- Check the skin several times a day, assessing for any areas of skin change: remember, 2 hourly for high-risk patients, 4 hourly for medium risk and daily for low risk.
- Keep the patient's skin dry from urine, sweat or wound leakage as this may lead to excoriation and skin breakdown.
- Keep the skin clean using a mild soap; highly scented soaps may cause skin dryness.
- Protect the skin over bony areas.
- If necessary, use special equipment and pads as part of pressure-relief management.
- Moisturise regularly using non-alcohol-based lotions, to keep the skin supple.
- Pat the skin dry; do not rub it when drying with a towel because this may cause skin damage by friction.

There are several ideal opportunities that you can take to check your patient's skin:

- when you are moving or turning your patient,
- when you are washing or bathing your patient,
- when you are assisting with dressing,
- when fitting shoes, slippers or socks,
- when assisting when toileting,
- when performing continence care.

NUTRITION

Pressure ulcer management includes providing a healthy balanced diet. Patients with pressure ulcers may need to be referred to a dietician for supplementary nutritional support.

What to eat:

- protein: for healing and the immune system (meat, eggs, lentils, yoghurt, etc.),
- carbohydrates: for energy, and also fibre to reduce constipation (bread, rice, pasta, potatoes, etc.),
- fats (in moderation): aid vitamin absorption.

EPUAP CLASSIFICATION SYSTEM

Pressure ulcers are classified according to their severity. Once present, the most commonly used scale is the EPUAP grading system (EPUAP 2003), also known as the EPUAP scale.

Grade	Assessment
1	Non-blanching erythema of intact skin. Discolouration of the skin, warmth, oedema, induration or hardness may also be used as indicators, particularly on individuals with darker skin.
2	Partial-thickness skin loss involving epidermis, dermis or both. The ulcer is superficial and presents clinically as an abrasion or blister.
3	Full-thickness skin loss involving damage to or necrosis of subcutaneous tissue that may extend to but not through the underlying fascia.
4	Extensive destruction, tissue necrosis or damage to muscle, bone, or supporting structures with or without full thickness skin loss.

Adapted from European Pressure Ulcer Advisory Panel (1998).

From this information, the appropriate treatment plan can be implemented. As part of the ongoing care, once a pressure ulcer has been identified documentation should include:

- cause of ulcer (if known),
- site/location of ulcer,
- size/dimensions of ulcer,
- grade of ulcer,
- exudate amount and type,
- whether ulcer has become infected,
- pain,
- wound appearance,
- description of surrounding skin,
- undermining/tracking (sinus or fistula),
- odour,
- multidisciplinary team involvement.

Assessment should be supported by photography and/or tracings to record the dimensions of the pressure ulcer, and its depth measured using a sterile probe.

The tissue-viability team will then create the optimum wound-healing management strategy according to the patient's individual needs using dressings such as hydrocolloids, hydrogels, hydrofibres, foams, films, alginates and/or soft silicones.

PRESSURE ULCER RISK ASSESSMENT TOOL

Many clinical areas use documentation similar to the Daily Pressure Ulcer Risk Assessment Tool (Figure 5.1), which incorporates pressure ulcer risk factors. These assessments should be undertaken on admission and the frequency of continued skin assessment may be conducted 2 hourly, 4 hourly or on a daily basis, depending on the individual needs. This frequency can be changed at any time as dictated by the patient's condition.

Daily Pressure Ulcer Risk Assessment Tool

North Bristol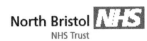
NHS Trust

Small Addressograph:

Patient surname:

First name:

Hospital no.:

Ward: Date:

Transferred to ward: Transfer date:

- **Risk assessment must be completed within 6 hours of admission**
- **Must be re-assessed daily as a minimum.**
- **Re-assess if clinical condition changes / transferred to other wards**

Daily risk factors (NICE guidance CG29 2005)

Please tick (✓) each day if risk factors are present and complete the daily record of risk assessment below:

	Date	Date	Date	Date		SKIN check frequency	Recommended equipment & therapy
High Risk							
Existing pressure ulcer or previous history of pressure ulcers						**SKIN check** **2 HOURLY** **Minimum** Discuss pressure ulcer prevention with patient/ relative - MDT consideration	Electric profiling bed frame with dynamic replacement mattress. Dynamic mattress may vary: Autologic, Nimbus 2 or Nimbus 3. Repose – add foot protectors (if necessary)
Reduced responsiveness to verbal or painful stimulus					If any factors present		
Pain – that reduces mobility							
Epidural							
Skin moist nearly all of the time (e.g. skin moist despite containment interventions for incontinence)							
Confined to bed or chair most of the time							
Makes only occasional or no change in position without assistance						Registered nursing staff must use their own clinical judgement to step down from dynamic mattresses if it is compromising patient rehabilitation. These recommendations are guidance only. Deviation from care must be recorded on page 4.	
Eating less than 1/2 of meals							
Needs moderate to maximum assistance in moving with high risk of friction against surface							
Clinical obesity - BMI >40							
Medium Risk							
Sensory impairment					If any factors present and none higher	**SKIN check** **4 HOURLY** **Minimum** Discuss pressure ulcer prevention with patient/ relative - MDT consideration.	Electric profiling bed frame and pressure reducing static mattress. Repose – add foot protectors (if necessary) Encourage mobility. Ensure seating assessed to reflect patient needs. Regular skin checks required.
Skin often moist (e.g. incontinent but containment interventions satisfactory)							
Walks occasionally							
Mobility limited							
Generally eats only half of any meal							
Needs some assistance to move with some contact against surface							
Vascular disease							
Severe chronic or palliative illness							
Low Risk							
Steroids					If any factors present and none higher	**SKIN check** **DAILY** **Minimum** Discuss skin care with patient/ relative - MDT consideration	Static bed frame and pressure reducing static mattress e.g. softform / pentaflex
No sensory deficit to pain							
Skin rarely moist							
Walks frequently							
No limitation in mobility							
Moves in bed & chair independently – able to lift self over surface with low friction risk							
Eats most of every meal							

Daily record of risk assessment

Date:	Time:	Risk level (tick):			Staff name:		Designation (tick): * must be countersigned				
		Low	Medium	High	Signature:	PRINT NAME:	HCA*	AP*	RGN / RGM	AHP	Student Nurse*

Figure 5.1 Daily Pressure Ulcer Risk Assessment Tool documentation. Permission to reproduce this image is granted by North Bristol NHS Trust and University Hospitals Bristol NHS Foundation Trust.

TEST YOUR KNOWLEDGE

Using the Daily Pressure Ulcer Risk Assessment Tool documentation (Figure 5.1), how often should the skin be checked according to these risk factors on the following 6 patients?

1   Walks frequently
2   Vascular disease
3   Eats most of every meal
4   Pain, which reduces mobility
5   Limited mobility
6   Clinical obesity (body mass index >40 kg/m^2)

KEY POINTS

- Pressure ulcer assessment.
- Pressure ulcer risk factors.
- Skin care.
- European Pressure Ulcer Advisory Panel classification system.
- Daily Pressure Ulcer Risk Assessment Tool documentation.

Bibliography

Anderson, I. (2012) Multidimensional leg ulcer assessment. *Nursing Times* 108(13), 17–20.

Bennett, G., Dealey, C. and Posnett, J. (2004) The cost of pressure ulcers in the UK. *Age and Aging* 33, 230–235.

Department of Health (2001) *The Essence of Care; Patient-focused Benchmarking for Health Care Practitioners.* The Stationery Office, London.

European Pressure Ulcer Advisory Panel (1998) *Pressure Ulcer Prevention and Treatment Guidelines.* www.epuap.org.uk

European Pressure Ulcer Advisory Panel (2003) Guidelines on the role of nutrition in pressure ulcer prevention and management. *EPUAP Review* 5(2), 45–76.

European Pressure Ulcer Advisory Panel and National Pressure Ulcer Advisory Panel (2009) *Pressure Ulcer Prevention - Quick Reference Guide.* www.npuap .org/wp-content/uploads/2012/02/Final_Quick_Prevention_for_web_2010.pdf.

National Institute for Clinical Excellence (2001) *Pressure Ulcer risk Assessment and Prevention.* National Institute for Clinical Excellence, London.

National Institute for Clinical Excellence (2003) *Clinical Guideline 7; Pressure Ulcer Prevention.* National Institute for Clinical Excellence, London.

National Institute for Clinical Excellence (2005) *The Prevention and Treatment of Pressure Ulcers.* National Institute for Clinical Excellence, London.

Royal College of Nursing (2006) *The Nursing Management of Patients with Venous Leg Ulcers.* Tinyurl.com/RCN-venous.

Website

Homepage for the Waterlow risk assessment tool: www.judy-waterlow.co.uk

Chapter 6
. . . .
PATIENT SAFETY

Care Skills for Nurses, First Edition. Claire Boyd
© 2014 John Wiley & Sons, Ltd. Published 2014 by John Wiley & Sons, Ltd.

LEARNING OUTCOMES

By the end of this chapter you will have an understanding of patient safety issues.

Patients come into hospital, in the main, to be made better. However, statistics tell us that many of these patients (11%) experience an adverse event during their hospital stay, with one third of these events leading to a severe disability or even death. Some 50% of these occurrences are avoidable (National Patient Safety Agency 2007a). There is little wonder, then, that much emphasis has been placed on reducing these shocking statistics. Three main categories have came to light while exploring these failures of care in the healthcare system:

1 failure to recognise,
2 failure to respond,
3 failure to communicate.

In other words, we were not noticing when our patients have deteriorated, not acting with enough speed when a problem is seen and not reporting our concerns to senior staff quickly enough. From these failures of care lessons have been learned and services improved, especially concerning patient safety matters. In the above categories much has been implemented to improve services, and you can see which of the Safer Patient Initiatives (also known as SPIs) fit into which category:

1 failure to recognise: Early Warning Scores (or EWS), incorporated into observation charts,
2 failure to respond: new observation charts (escalation measures),
3 failure to communicate: SBAR communication tool, or Situation, Background, Assessment, Recommendation.

SAFETY BRIEFINGS

Facts and figures are collected from daily, weekly and monthly audits. Such audits look at the frequency of things like cardiac arrests, patients at risk of falling, peripheral-line infections, drug errors and raised EWS. Data from these audits then go to the NHS Audit Department so that improvements can be made. From this we can improve services by highlighting concerns and identifying themes within clinical areas and directorates.

PATIENT SAFETY

Patient safety covers many areas, such as:

- Early Warning Scores (EWS),
- observation charts,
- escalation measures,
- SBAR communication,
- falls prevention,
- safety briefings.

Most of these topics are covered in *Clinical Skills for Nurses* from the Student Survival Skills Series (Boyd 2013), but one area that is not touched on is falls prevention. That is explored in this chapter.

FALLS PREVENTION

First let's start by looking at some of the annual statistics reported by the National Patient Safety Agency (2010):

- 200 000 falls were reported in acute hospitals in England and Wales,
- more than 36 000 falls were reported in mental health units,
- finally, there were 38 000 falls in community hospitals.

A significant number of these falls result in death or injury, including more than 800 hip fractures and more than 500 other fractures (National Patient Safety Agency 2010).

Let's look at some more statistics:

- falls account for 20% of hospital admissions,
- falls account for 20 million bed days per year,
- 40% of care home admissions are as a result of a fall,
- 50% of people who suffer a hip fracture as a result of a fall can no longer live independently,
- 20% of older people who suffer a hip fracture as a result of a fall die within 6 months.

Financially, it has been estimated that in-patient falls cost an estimated £15 000 000 a year for immediate treatment, with the costs during the ensuing rehabilitation and social care being even greater. But what about the human cost? Lack of mobility and pain can have devastating psychological effects on well-being. In addition, patients admitted after a fall are more vulnerable due to their falls history, with analgesia and/or sedation and disorientation exacerbating the problem still further.

Falls are not an inevitable part of ageing! But let's look at some of the implications of falls in older people:

- physical injuries,
- loss of independence,
- psychological: fear of falling,
- social impact,
- carer impact,
- cost to services.

FALLS AT HOME

Statistics tell us that falls do not only occur in the hospital setting: one third of adults over 65, and living at home, will experience at least one fall a year, rising to half of adults over 80 who are either at home or in residential care. The very fear of falling, with loss of confidence, has made many elderly 'prisoners in their own homes' (BBC 2012).

Making changes at home can help to prevent falls, such as:

- ensuring that rooms are well-lit,
- making sure the environment is clutter free,
- laying non-slip mats and rugs.

IN-PATIENT FALLS

Initiatives are also being devised to reduce in-patient falls, but we first need to start by looking at the main individual risk factors.

Question 6.1   What do you think are six of the main individual risk factors for in-patient falls?

Many of these factors can be addressed by assessment and treatment, such as by treating the urinary problems, adjusting the medication and, if able, providing walking aids.

Question 6.2   Why do older people fall? List five environmental risk factors that you think could make an older person more likely to fall while in hospital.

REDUCING PATIENT FALLS

To reduce patient falls, first and foremost we need to find the **cause**.

- Falls as a presentation to hospital or during admission may indicate acute illness (such as an infection), or may be due to a more chronic condition (such as previous strokes, Parkinson's disease or memory problems).
- Also, remember: if the person says they blacked out or think they might have blacked out it is very important that they see a doctor, as this could be to do with their heart.
- The patient may need to have clinical investigations.
- Medicines need to be reviewed.

- Exercise can help people keep fit and if they need specific exercises for balance they might see a physiotherapist or go to an exercise and balance group.
- If there are hazards around the home an occupational therapist can give advice, and home-improvement agencies like Care and Repair can help with putting up rails, tacking down loose carpets and other tasks in the home.
- In some areas Age Concern can give lists of approved contractors to help with jobs to make the home safe.

It is important when talking to older people about falls prevention that we empower them to take responsibility for their own lifestyle. We should present falls prevention in a positive light, as a way to retain independence and maintain quality of life.

Many areas now have falls services with a falls co-ordinator, to whom the patient can be referred.

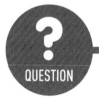

Question 6.3   What interventions we can offer to minimise the risk of falls?

There are many interventions that can be put in place to minimise the risk of falls in hospital:

- ensuring the patient has appropriate, well-fitting footwear,
- ensuring the patient has a call bell within reach to contact staff for assistance,
- ensuring that glasses are on the ward and clean, and that hearing aids are on the ward and work,
- ensuring that any reported change in vision is reviewed by a doctor,
- offering regular toileting assistance to those with frequency and continence issues,

- ensuring that the bedside is free from clutter,
- using a low bed in circumstances when the patient is at risk of rolling/climbing out of bed and then falling.

FOOTWEAR

Footwear needs to be sturdy and well-fitting. Unsafe footwear may include:

- bare feet,
- socks only,
- anti-embolic stockings,
- bandages or dressings only,
- shoes/slippers that are visibly too big,
- shoes/slippers that are visibly too small,
- laces undone or missing,
- worn shoes with squashed backs,
- novelty slippers,
- backless shoes or slippers,
- foam disposable slippers,
- high-heeled shoes.

IN VERY HIGH-RISK PATIENTS

For very high-risk patients an intervention called **intentional rounding** has been shown to reduce the risk of falls in hospital. This requires nursing staff to observe a patient every hour, asking questions and offering help, in a set order, about:

- toileting,
- pain,
- confusion,
- comfort/position,
- offering a drink,
- reminding the patient about the call bell/ensuring it is in reach,
- checking bed height,
- checking that rails are down,
- asking whether anything else is needed.

Figure 6.1 shows an example of the documentation for this type of intervention.

8/7/2011

North Bristol NHS
NHS Trust

Intentional Rounding Checklist Tool for Falls

Name

Hospital Number — Falls leaflet given ☐ Continence checked Supervision for toileting documented in notes

DOB — Doctors asked to review medication Referral made to physiotherapy Vision checked ☐

Ward — **Round every 1 hr for High risk 2 hr for Medium risk** (Circle times below and initial after each round)

Date: Time:	8 am	9 am	10 am	11 am	12 n	1 pm	2 pm	3 pm	4 pm	5 pm	6 pm	7 pm	8 pm	9 pm	10 pm	11 pm	12 mn	1 am	2 am	3 am	4 am	5 am	6 am	7 am
ARE YOU COMFORTABLE? Re-positioned 2 hourly																								
DO YOU NEED THE TOILET?																								
DO YOU HAVE ANY PAIN?																								
Orientated= O (please indicate) confused =C asleep=A																								
WOULD YOU LIKE A DRINK? Fluids offered																								
Call bell within reach **IF YOU NEED ME, PLEASE PRESS THIS BUTTON.**																								
Bed rails down/bed lowest position																								
Footwear checked																								
IS THERE ANYTHING ELSE I CAN DO? I HAVE THE TIME																								

Figure 6.1 Intentional Rounding Checklist Tool For Falls. Permission to reproduce this image is granted by North Bristol NHS Trust and University Hospitals Bristol NHS Foundation Trust.

THE MULTIDISCIPLINARY TEAM

Minimise the risk of falls in high-risk patients involve the multidisciplinary team, which includes:

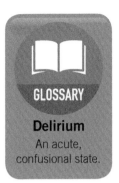

GLOSSARY

Delirium
An acute,
confusional state.

- assessment by a physiotherapist and occupational therapist,
- review of medication by a pharmacist or doctor,
- continence assessment if the patient has urinary or bowel problems,
- visual assessment by a doctor if there are newly reported problems with vision,
- memory assessment by a doctor if the patient is confused.

FALLS AND DELIRIUM

Part of the Safer Patient Initiatives in preventing falls includes recognising and managing delirium. In other words, spotting and treating the condition. Six of the most common causes of delirium are known by the acronym PINCH ME. Look at Table 6.1 to find out what this means.

Table 6.1 Recognising and managing delirium

Delirium =	Acute confusion is a sign that someone is physically unwell
1 Spot it	Sudden change in behaviour More confused over the past few hours or days Confusion varies at different times of the day Difficulty in following a conversation Rambling and jumping from topic to topic More sleepy or more agitated than usual If any answers are 'Yes' it could be delirium. If in doubt, check it out!
2 Treat it	Remember the six common causes of delirium: PINCH ME! PINCH ME = Pain, Infection, Constipation, Hydration, Medication, Environment

(continued)

Table 6.1 *(Continued)*

3 Stop!	*Explanation and reassurance:* introduce yourself and explain what you are doing. Be calm and patient, avoid being confrontational.
	Reorientation: remind the person of the time, date or season. Set clocks and calendars to the right time and date. Turn down noisy TVs and radios.
	Look after physical needs: drinking, eating, toileting, sleep time, prevent falls. Check for signs of infection or pain.

Permission to reproduce this table is granted by North Bristol NHS Trust and University Hospitals Bristol NHS Foundation Trust.

FALLS RISK ASSESSMENT

Patients being admitted to hospital should have a falls risk assessment performed. The documentation should be completed within 6 hours of admission, after a move to a new ward and if the patient's condition changes; for example, if the patient becomes unwell or has a fall. This risk assessment tool should be re-assessed on a weekly basis. Student nurses (and others) should familiarise themselves with the necessary paperwork. Figures 6.2 and 6.3 show examples of some of this documentation.

BEDRAILS

Bedrails (not to be called 'cot sides' as this is very demeaning to adult patients) are an effective safety tool, used to reduce the risk of falls from bed. Bedrails should not be used with acutely confused patients.

Before using, three questions should be asked.

1   Is the patient likely to fall from bed?
2   Is the bedrail the best solution?
3   Are there alternatives (e.g. a low bed)?

If used inappropriately bedrails can lead to serious injury or even death due to:

- entrapment,
- climbing over and falling to the floor.

| Forename(s): |
| Surname: |
| Hospital No: |
| DOB: |

Every Shift Falls Prevention Care Plan

To be completed for lower risk patients

North Bristol **NHS**
NHS Trust

Ward:
Date:

Please record date, signature and A (= Achieved) or V (=Variance) and record overleaf
If patient is Medium or High Risk please use Intentional Rounding Care Plan

Review every prevention intervention every shift	Date			Date			Date			Date			Date			Date			Date		
	E	L	N	E	L	N	E	L	N	E	L	N	E	L	N	E	L	N	E	L	N
Environment (Clutter removed? Extra lighting? e.g. bedside lamp left on overnight, night light in toilet. Right place on ward? e.g. Close to the nurses station, close to the toilet, quietest area)																					
Call bell (remind to use, ensure in reach, consider alternatives if unable to recall use of call bell, e.g. brass bell, move bed in sight of nurse station)																					
Bed rails (use according to assessment, ensure the bed is kept at the lowest height at all times)																					
Toileting (is Falls Risk associated with patient's need to use toilet? Frequency? Urgency? Urine Specimen? Does the patient's bed need to be nearer the toilet? Is the patient safe to leave alone behind curtains or in bathroom?)																					
Footwear (being worn by patient? Secure fit? Ask relatives to supply safer replacement if required? Consider slipper socks at night)																					
Glasses/hearing aid (on ward? In reach? Has the patient's vision changed? Ask doctor to assess acuity)																					
Medications (review any sedating drugs with pharmacist/doctor e.g. anti-depressants, sleeping tablets, sedation, anti-psychotics)																					
Confusion (if new, get doctor to medically assess cognition. Does the patient require extra supervision/Intentional Rounding?)																					
MDT (Is the MDT aware of the falls risk? Has this patient been flagged at the safety briefing?																					
If above completed by HCA trained nurse to countersign																					

SES.v4.05/10/2011

Figure 6.2 *(continued)*

Date & time	Variance record	Signature
	Does patient require Supervision for toileting No Yes	
	Document details below:	

Figure 6.2 Falls Prevention Care Plan. Permission to reproduce this image is granted by North Bristol NHS Trust and University Hospitals Bristol NHS Foundation Trust.

For this reason, bedrails should be used *only* after a full bedrail assessment. Figure 6.4 shows an example of this documentation.

USING AN ULTRA-LOW BED

Using ultra-low beds can help to prevent harm from falls, particularly for patients with delirium who are at risk of falling out of bed but who cannot be given bedrails as they may try to climb over them. However, ultra-low beds need to be used safely and appropriately.

The National Patient Safety Agency (2007b) identified a series of incidents related to incorrect use of ultra-low beds:

- injuries from floor-level furniture or fittings such as radiators, pipes or lockers (including one serious burn),
- ultra-low beds placed close to a wall but not flush with it, creating the potential for asphyxia entrapment if the patient slipped between the side of the mattress and the wall,
- ultra-low beds left at working height in error, leading to falls from height,
- patients who appeared to have tripped over crash mats used beside the ultra-low bed (including three fractured hips).

North Bristol **NHS**
NHS Trust

Falls Risk Assessment Tool

Patient Name:	Hospital no:	Ward:	Date:

- **Patient risk assessment must be completed on admission and weekly as a minimum.**
- **If patient's clinical condition changes or changes ward, please reassess.**
- **Give NBT Patient Falls Prevention leaflet to all patients**

Addressograph:

Risk Factors
Please tick if any of the risk factors are present below:

HIGH RISK

Date
Acute confusion/delirium
Fall in hospital this admission
Attempting to stand or walk unaided when not safe to do so
Using your clinical judgment, the patient would benefit from intentional rounding

If any factors present → Intentional Rounding Minimum **HOURLY**

MEDIUM RISK

Fall as the presenting complaint for admission
Chronic confusion or dementia
Unsteady when walking/turning
Prescribed sedative medication
Under influence or withdrawing from alcohol/drugs
The multi-disciplinary team feels the patient is at risk of falling

If **3 factors or above** present, and **none** higher → Complete **Intentional Rounding** Minimum **2 HOURLY**

If **less than 3 factors** present →

LOWER

Previous falls (not related to presentation or admission)
Any other concerns (previous fracture, post-operative)
Relatives anxious about falls

If **any** factors present, and **none** higher → Complete **Falls Care Plan EVERY SHIFT**

Minimal RISK

None of the above risk factors present

Re-assess **weekly** or if **change** in clinical **condition**

Weekly record of risk assessment:

Date	Time	Risk level (tick)				Staff name		Designation (tick)			
		Minimal risk	Lower	Medium	High	Signature	PRINT NAME	HCA*	Student nurse*	AP*	RGN

* **must be countersigned**

SES.v10.6/06/2011

13/12/2010

RVJ0804 lgd

Figure 6.3 Falls Risk Assessment Tool. Permission to reproduce this image is granted by North Bristol NHS Trust and University Hospitals Bristol NHS Foundation Trust.

North Bristol **NHS**

NHS Trust

ADULT PATIENT BEDRAIL RISK ASSESSMENT								
Directorate		Patient Details *(Affix label if available)*						
Ward								

The Falls Risk Assessment must be completed prior to completion of this bedrail assessment.

Staff should use the bedrail risk assessment in addition to their **professional judgement** to consider the risks and benefits for Individual patients.

RISK FACTOR Please record answers to these questions in box ✓=yes ✗=no	USE OF BEDRAILS	NOTES	Date Initial of Reviewer					
Patient is independently mobile	Bedrails not to be used	Check patient has not requested use of bedrails						
Patient **is likely to** attempt to get out of bed alone	Bedrails not to be used	Use height adjustable bed to suit patients requirements						
Patient has previously attempted to climb over bedrails	Bedrails not to be used	Consider use of low height bed						
Patient has uncontrolled limb movements / restless/ significantly confused	Bedrails not to be used	Consider use of low height bed						
Patient has difficulty rolling over in bed	Bedrails not to be used							
Patient **is not likely to** attempt to get out of bed alone	**Consider use of Bedrails**	Optional use of protective bedrail bumpers						
Patient has disruption to their spatial or visual awareness	**Consider use of Bedrails**	Optional use of protective bedrail bumpers						
Patient has a fear of falling out of bed whilst asleep	**Consider use of Bedrails**	Ensure bedrails are securely fitted in matching pairs, and in good working order						
Patient is recovering from an anaesthetic	**Bedrails to be used**	Ensure bedrails are securely fitted in matching pairs, and in good working order						
Patient has requested bedrails or uses bedrails at home	**Bedrails to be used**	Ensure bedrails are securely fitted in matching pairs, and in good working order						
Patient is unconscious or completely immobile	**Bedrails to be used**	Ensure bedrails are securely fitted in matching pairs, and in good working order						
	Please put bed rail sign above the bed	**BED RAILS USED (tick and initial)**						
		BED RAILS NOT USED (tick and initial)						

If risk factors conflict e.g. Patient is independently mobile and the patient has requested bedrails, or uses bedrails at home, staff need to use their **professional judgement** to consider the risks and benefits for individual patients and document.

Consideration should be given to other control measures when completing this assessment.

Report any faulty bed rails to the Huntleigh Equipment Library for repair as soon as possible

Figure 6.4 *(continued)*

Date & time	Variance record	Signature

Figure 6.4 Adult Patient Bedrail Risk Assessment. Permission to reproduce this image is granted by North Bristol NHS Trust and University Hospitals Bristol NHS Foundation Trust.

VERY HIGH-RISK PATIENTS

Not all patients' risk can be adequately reduced, but we can still implement certain measures, such as:

- alerting all colleagues to the patient's high level of risk,
- assessing the risk and documenting any actions that have been taken,
- 'specialling' the patient, meaning that 1:1 nursing will be implemented, if agreed,
- documenting changes on a daily basis.

WHAT TO DO IF A PATIENT FALLS

If a patient falls, the following actions need to be performed:
- assess the patient for injury,
- make regular observations, including neurological observations (using the Glasgow Coma Scale; see chapter 10 of Clinical Skills for Nurses, Boyd 2012),
- carry out a medical review,
- be aware of the potential for cerebral bleeding in patients who are being given anticoagulants,
- discuss risks with the patient and inform their relatives,
- re-assess the patient's falls risk and review measures to prevent further falls,
- complete all documentation, including any post-falls actions forms and incident forms.

Neurological observations should be performed if there is any suspicion of a head injury. Usual recording intervals are:

- quarter hourly for the first 2 hours,
- half hourly for 2 hours,
- hourly for 2 hours,
- 2 hourly for 4 hours,
- then 4 hourly until 24 hours post-fall.

TEST YOUR KNOWLEDGE

1 What were the three main categories identified as to why 11% of patients experience an adverse event during their hospital stay, and what strategies have been put in place to improve services?
2 How many patients falls, according to the National Patient Safety Agency (2010), are reported in mental health units?
3 What do you think are the main implications of falls in older people?
4 What is intentional rounding?
5 How can inappropriately used bedrails lead to serious injury or even death?
6 Six of the common causes of delirium are known by the phrase PINCH ME: what does it stand for?

KEY POINTS

- Patient safety topics.
- Falls risk factors.
- Intentional rounding.
- Falls and delirium.
- Bedrail and falls risk assessment tools.

Bibliography

Baba-Akbari, A., Sheldon, T.A., Cracknell, A. and Turnbull, A. (2007) Patient safety incidents in an NHS hospital. *British Medical Journal* 334, 79.

BBC (2012) Elderly people staying at home for fear of falling. 31 October. www.bbc
.co.uk/news/health-20138731.

Boyd, C. (2013) *Clinical Skills for Nurses*. Wiley Blackwell, Oxford.

Department of Health (2001) *National Service Framework for Older Adults*. Standard
6. tinyurl.com/dh-NSFOlderAdults.

Heaton, C. (2012) Creating a protocol to reduce inpatient falls. *Nursing Times*
108(12), 16–18.

National Institute for Clinical Excellence (2004) *The Assessment and Prevention of
Falls in Older People*. www.nice.org.uk/CG21.

National Patient Safety Agency (2007a) *Safer Care for the Acutely Ill Patient:
Learning from Serious Incidents*. National Patient Safety Agency, London.

National Patient Safety Agency (2007b) *Using Bedrails Safely and Effectively*.
tinyurl.com/NPSA-Bedrails.

National Patient Safety Agency (2010) *Slips, Trips and Falls in Hospital: Data
Update*. tinyuri.com/NPSA-SlipsFalls.

NHS Institute for Innovation and Improvement (2010) *High Impact Changes
for Nursing and Midwifery: the Essential Collection*. http://webarchive.
nationalarchives.gov.uk/20100702175948/http://www.institute.nhs.uk/images//
stories/Building_Capability/HIA/NHSI%20High%20Impact%20Actions.pdf.

Oliver, D., Healy, F. and Haines, T.P. (2010) Preventing falls and fall-related injuries
in hospitals. *Clinics in Geriatric Medicine* 26(4), 645–692.

Vincent, C., Neale, G. and Woloshynowych, M. (2001) Adverse events in British
hospitals. *British Medical Journal* 322, 517–519.

Chapter 7
. . . .
STOMA CARE

Care Skills for Nurses, First Edition. Claire Boyd
© 2014 John Wiley & Sons, Ltd. Published 2014 by John Wiley & Sons, Ltd.

LEARNING OUTCOMES

By the end of this chapter you will have an understanding of the theory and practice of providing nursing care to individuals with colostomies, ileostomies and urostomies.

Before we look at digestive and renal stomas, we first need to revisit the basic normal anatomy and physiology of these systems.

THE DIGESTIVE SYSTEM

The human digestive system, simplified, is a complex series of organs and glands that process the food that we eat by breaking them down into smaller molecules. The digestive process begins in the mouth by the action of salivary enzymes breaking down carbohydrates in our food. The food that we eat forms a bolus which, when swallowed, travels along the oesophagus into the stomach by a series of wave-like motions (called peristalsis). Once in the stomach, the food is churned around, partly digested, and bathed in gastric acid to produce chyme.

Food then enters the duodenum, the first part of the small intestine, travels to the jejunum and then the ileum (the final part of the small intestine). All the while, pancreatic enzymes, bile (from the gall bladder) and enzymes produced by the inner wall of the small intestine continue the process of food breakdown (see Figure 7.1).

Food then passes into the large intestine through the caecum, where water and electrolytes are removed from the food. Digestive bacteria such as *Bacteroides, Lactobacillus acidophilus, Escherichia coli* and *Klebsiella* assist in the digestive process. Food travels up into the ascending colon, along the transverse colon and down the descending colon into the sigmoid colon (part of the large intestine between the descending colon and the rectum). Solid waste is then stored in the rectum until it is excreted from the anus.

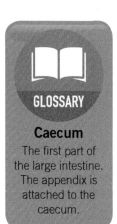

GLOSSARY

Caecum
The first part of the large intestine. The appendix is attached to the caecum.

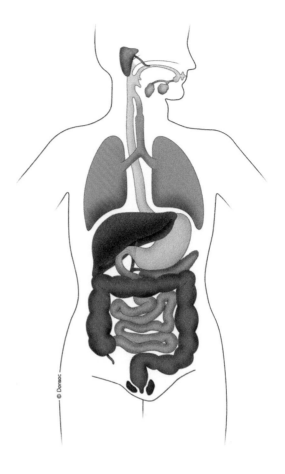

Figure 7.1 The human digestive system. Permission to use this image has kindly been given by Dansac Limited.

THE RENAL SYSTEM

Urine is made in the kidneys and is propelled into the bladder via two tubes, called ureters. Urine is then stored in the bladder, which passively expands to receive the urine. The bladder is composed of interlaced smooth muscle, known as the detrusor muscle. Two sphincters control the bladder outlet: the internal sphincter (controlled by the

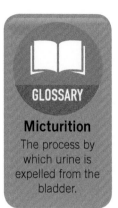

Micturition
The process by
which urine is
expelled from the
bladder.

autonomic nervous system) and the external sphincter (under voluntary control). As the bladder expands and pressure on the sphincters increases, the ureters are compressed, stopping any backflow of urine. Stretch receptors in the detrusor muscle signal that we need to void (pass urine), and the internal sphincter opens. The external sphinter then relaxes and micturition occurs.

WHAT IS A STOMA?

A *stoma* is a generic term for 'orifice' or 'mouth' in Greek. An artificial opening or passageway for faeces to be expelled from the small intestine (also known as the small bowel), through the muscle and out through the skin, is known as an **ileostomy**. A similar artificial opening or passageway from the large intestine (also known as the large bowel) is known as a **colostomy**.

Faeces have now been diverted and will not be expelled through the rectum and anus, but out through the stomal opening. As the faeces travel along the intestine they change, and the matter should generally become more formed as it passes through the bowel. Faeces from an ileostomy are more liquid and have a stronger odour due to the presence of the enzymes involved with food breakdown. In a colostomy the faeces are more formed, being more solid, as they have undergone more of the digestive process.

A stoma in the renal system is called a urinary diversion; also known as a **urostomy**. This is because urine is diverted away from the bladder. Other types of renal stoma are the **ileal conduit** and **nephrostomy**.

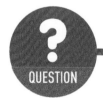

Question 7.1 What is an ileal conduit and what is a nephrostomy?

After surgery for a colostomy, ileostomy or urostomy the sphincter muscles are bypassed. There is no control over bowel movement and a collection device must be worn.

STOMAL APPEARANCE

The stoma itself should be warm, moist and red to dark pink in colour (like cheek mucosa). Patients sometimes call the stoma a 'bud' or 'strawberry' due to its colour and shape. This bud is very vascular, meaning that it will bleed profusely if cut. However, the patient will not feel this as the intestine has no nerve endings. The skin around this bud is known as the peristomal skin and will feel pain if the skin becomes damaged in any way.

Regardless of the type of surgery – bowel or renal – patients are referred to a specialised stoma care nurse who will advise and support the patient.

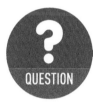

QUESTION

Question 7.2   Fill in the missing words:

Bowel stomas:
Large bowel diversion =
Small bowel diversion =

Renal stomas:
Urinary diversion =

REASONS FOR STOMA SURGERY

For a variety of reasons stoma surgery may be permanent or 'reversible'. It may be carried out for many medical conditions, including:

* irritable bowel syndrome (bowel),
* ulcerated colitis (bowel),
* cancer (bowel or urinary),
* diverticulitis or Crohn's disease (bowel),
* trauma (bowel or urinary),
* neurological damage (urinary or bowel),
* cancer of the pelvis (urinary or bowel),
* congenital disorder (urinary or bowel).

A reversible procedure is where the two cut ends are reattached, with any damaged or diseased area cut out. Not all patients are able to undergo a reversal operation.

DRAINAGE DEVICES

As the bodily waste (faecal matter or urine) now travels out of the body via the stoma, a collection device will need to be placed at the end of the stoma and attached to the body. Figure 7.2 shows an ileostomy drainage device attached to the skin.

Pouches, Flanges and Wafers

There are various types of collection device. There are two main types of pouch:

- **single use:** used when the skin is in good condition (see Figure 7.3),
- **drainable:** changed every 4–5 days, or sooner if outside of bag becomes soiled (see Figure 7.4).

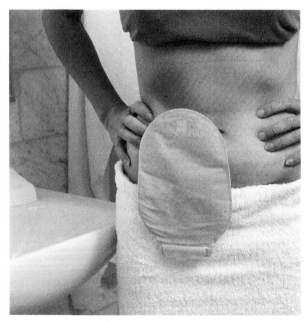

Figure 7.2 Ileostomy stoma device. Permission to use this image has kindly been given by Dansac Limited.

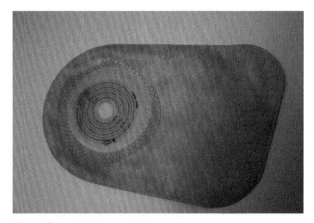

Figure 7.3 A single-use drainage bag.

Urostomy drainage systems have taps at the bottom of the bag, much like urinary catheter drainage bags, to empty the contents.

Pouches can be applied directly to the skin or used with a device known as a flange, onto which the bag can be attached and detached as required. The flange can remain in place for 4–5 days (see Figure 7.5).

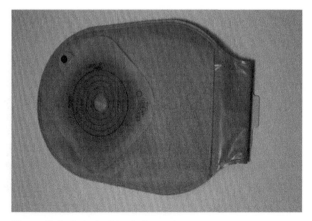

Figure 7.4 A drainable drainage bag.

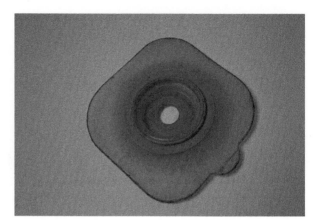

Figure 7.5 A flange.

Pouches may have Velcro or clips to keep the contents in the bag, which can be undone or removed to empty the contents. Digestive stomas may also be covered with a device known as a 'wafer' or 'plaster' which may be used if the individual wishes to go swimming or partake in sexual intercourse. Afterwards the wafer can be removed and a drainage device then re-applied (see Figure 7.6).

Stomas can be budded, flat, oval or round and stoma drainage systems can be convex or concave depending

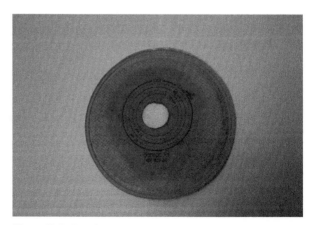

Figure 7.6 A wafer.

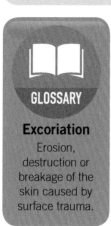

GLOSSARY

Excoriation

Erosion, destruction or breakage of the skin caused by surface trauma.

on the bud (whether an 'innie' or an 'outie'). When preparing a new bag for attachment the stoma is measured with a measuring gauge and the hole on the bag is cut to size after softening any sharp edges. For example, if the measuring gauge shows that the stoma is 30 mm, then the bag gets cut to this size. The bag has different sizes printed on it to show where to cut for a particular size. A stoma can change in size as a result of weight gain or loss. The pouch should be warmed in the hands first to enable better bag adhesion and pliability. Patients who have had their stomas for many years tend not to change the stoma size to a great degree so these patients may well receive pre-cut bags by prescription.

SKIN CONDITION

The peristomal skin should be healthy. If it becomes red, sore or excoriated you must report it immediately to the nurse in charge or district nurse as appropriate. Only specialised products can be applied to the peristomal skin, as products like Sudocreme do not allow the drainage bag to stick to the skin. The registered nurse overseeing your practice may wish the patient to be referred to a specialised stoma care nurse.

BODY IMAGE

Clients and patients may be worried about their body image. They may ask you for advice regarding sexual activity and my advice was always 'Go for it'! It is best to empty the drainage device before you start. An accident with a burst drainage bag could have very unpleasant results.

It is always best to encourage the individual to empty their own drainage bags as a means of promoting self care. However, not all clients have the cognitive function or dexterity to perform this activity. In such cases the carer must never show any revulsion when assisting with stoma or renal drainage, as this can adversely affect a patient's psychological well-being.

CHANGING A STOMA BAG

Drainage bags should be emptied into a lavatory or a container prior to removal. If able, get the patient to sit as far back on the toilet seat as possible and empty the contents down the lavatory. Alternatively, the patient may prefer to stand or kneel, whichever is easiest.

When the bag has been emptied it can be removed, very gently, while holding the skin taut. The peristomal area will need to be cleaned with soap and water and dried well. A new drainage device can be applied after being measured using a measuring gauge and cut to size for a tight fit. Full personal protective equipment should be worn – apron and gloves – if you are carrying out this procedure.

DISPOSAL OF THE STOMA BAG

In a clinical setting the stoma bag should be disposed of in a clinical waste bag.

In the community the bag should be wrapped in a plastic bag and then wrapped in a second bag. It can then be disposed of in a household waste bin if the client does not have a dedicated waste bin. As already mentioned, the urine and faecal matter should be emptied down the toilet first as you cannot discard human waste with normal household waste.

ISSUES TO CONSIDER

After ileostomy surgery the patient may experience water and electrolyte loss, meaning that hydration must be well maintained to prevent dehydration. In addition, after any digestive ostomy surgery digestion and absorption of medicines may be affected. In such cases the patient will require a full review of their medicines.

Urinary tract infections are common in individuals who have undergone urostomy surgery. Preventive measures include drinking plenty of fluids and emptying the pouch regularly.

Certain foods, such as mushrooms, sweetcorn, dried fruit and tomato skins, may cause blockages in an ileostomy. These foods may need to be cut into smaller pieces during preparation.

TEST YOUR KNOWLEDGE

1 Name two types of urinary stoma.
2 What does peristomal skin mean?
3 Give four reasons why someone may require stoma surgery.
4 What should only specialised products be applied to the peristomal skin area?

KEY POINTS

- The digestive and renal systems.
- Different types of stoma.
- The appearance of a healthy stoma.
- The rationale for stoma surgery.
- Drainage devices.
- Peristomal skin condition.
- Body image after stoma surgery.
- Changing and disposal of drainage bags.
- Issues to consider after stoma surgery.

Bibliography

Bass, E.M., Del Pino, A., Tan, A. et al. (1997) Does preoperative stoma marking and education by the enterostomal therapist affect outcome? *Diseases of the Colon and Rectum* 40(94), 440–442.

Black, P. (1994) Stoma care: a practical approach. *Nursing Standard* 8(34), RCN Nurses' Update Learning Unit 045.

Black, P. (1997) Practical stoma care. *Nursing Standard* 11 (47), 49–53.

Black, P. (1998) Colostomy. *Professional Nurse* 13(12), 851–857.

Black, P. (2000) Practical stoma care. *Nursing Standard* 14(41), 47–55.

Black, P. (2004) Psychological, sexual and cultural issues for patients with a stoma. *British Journal of Nursing* 13(12), 692–697.

Borwell, B. (1994) Colostomies and their management. *Nursing Standard* 8(45), CE article 332.

Taylor, P. (2005) An introduction to stomas: reasons for their formation. *Nursing Times* 101(29), 63–64.

Thibodeau, G. and Patton, K.T. (2007) *Anatomy and Physiology*, 6th edn. Mosby Elsevier, St Louis, MO.

Willis, J. (1995) Stoma care principles and product type. *Nursing Times* 91(2), 43–45.

Wilson, M. (2008) Diarrhoea and its possible impact on skin health. *Nursing Times* 104(18), 49–52.

Wood, S. (1998) Nutrition and stoma patients. *Nursing Times* 94(48), 65–67.

Website

Homepage for a maker of stoma products: www.dansac.co.uk

Chapter 8

· · · · · · · · · · · · · · · · · · · ·

PERI-OPERATIVE CARE

Care Skills for Nurses, First Edition. Claire Boyd
© 2014 John Wiley & Sons, Ltd. Published 2014 by John Wiley & Sons, Ltd.

GLOSSARY

Elective surgery

Not necessary for the patient's survival, but expected to improve the patient's health.

Essential surgery

Necessary to prevent or remove a threat to the patient's life.

Emergency surgery

Necessary to be performed with minimal delay in the interest of the patient's survival.

WHAT IS PERI-OPERATIVE CARE?

Peri-operative care concerns three phases of the surgical procedure: when the patient is admitted to hospital for surgery, the surgery itself and the aftercare. These phases are known respectively as:

1   pre-operative,
2   intra-operative,
3   post-operative.

Operations may be categorised as minor or major. Patients may also require different types of anaesthesia, such as general anaesthetic (sometimes called GA), a regional block (such as a spinal block, epidural or nerve block) or a local anaesthetic. Patient aftercare will very much depend on the type of anaesthetic used. How we prepare our patients for the operating theatre varies greatly due to the variety of surgical procedures and whether the procedure is classified as elective, essential or emergency. Whichever type of surgery, the peri-operative period starts with the assessment of the patient in preparation for their surgery.

How involved a student nurse gets involved in the peri-operative process depends on what stage they are at in their nurse training.

PRE-ADMISSION ASSESSMENT

Some patients may attend a pre-admission clinic some time before their surgical procedure. It is here that the patient will undergo a full examination, have vital signs collected, undergo venepuncture, have MRSA screening performed and have a history taken to establish their fitness for the operation they require.

Question 8.1 What six vital signs, or observations, would you need to undertake for a pre-operative patient?

This assessment process can also provide the opportunity to check that the patient has been fully informed regarding their procedure and that consent is obtained. In short, the physical and psychological preparation begins here.

NURSING ASSESSMENT AND THE NURSING PROCESS

Once a patient is admitted to hospital an individualised care plan is prepared if it has not already been done during the pre-assessment clinic. This involves implementing the nursing process (Box 8.1).

Box 8.1   The nursing process

- Assessment
- Nursing diagnosis
- Planning
- Implementation
- Evaluation

The nursing process is a cyclical process. It is never static, as you will need to re-evaluate the whole process as the patient's condition changes.

During assessment the patient may need to be fitted for compression (anti-embolism) stockings used for the prevention of venous thromboembolism (VTE), including a DVT.

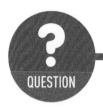

Question 8.2 What is a DVT?

It is recommended that patients wear compression stockings after surgery until their ability to move about has increased. Stockings prevent blood clots developing in the deep veins of the body, usually the legs. Patients may need to wear compression stockings even if they are undergoing surgery and being discharged from hospital on the same day. Patients may be more at risk of VTE if:

- mobility is expected to be significantly reduced for 3 or more days,
- the surgery lasts more than 90 minutes,
- the surgery lasts more than 60 minutes if the operation is on the pelvis or one of the legs.

PRE-OPERATIVE PREPARATION

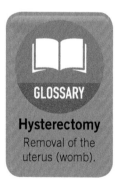

GLOSSARY

Hysterectomy
Removal of the uterus (womb).

Female patients will need to be asked, usually by the medic, whether there is a possibility of pregnancy or whether they are presently menstruating. If so you will need to make sure that she has a sanitary towel in place and not a tampon. Of course, this does not mean all female patients, as patients who are no longer of childbearing age or who have undergone a hysterectomy can be spared this question.

Consent will need to be checked and any investigations carried out, such as electrocardiogram (ECG) recording. All jewellery and cosmetics should be removed and wedding bands covered with hypoallergenic tape. Valuables should be placed in the hospital's custody and recorded according to hospital policy.

If the patient is undergoing urological or gynaecological surgery underwear will need to be removed. Cotton underwear may be worn otherwise. The patient should have a shower, or a bed bath, as close as possible to the planned time of the operation and premedication can then be administered, if prescribed, after the patient has been invited to pass urine.

The patient may require assistance to don their theatre gown and will need to have their anti-embolic stockings fitted correctly. It is a good idea to check that the patient is still wearing identification bracelets. Always ask the patient when they last had food and drink; document their answer. The patient will also need to be asked about dentures, which will need to be removed, and whether they have any dental crowns, bridge work or loose teeth. This information will need to be relayed to the anaesthetist.

Glasses and hearing aids can remain *in situ* until the last moment in the anaesthetic room, but contact lenses will need to be removed, as will any moveable prosthesis. If a local anaesthetic is being used then hearing aids may be retained if they do not interfere with the operation.

At this stage the pre-operative check list needs to be checked and all documentation gathered. The premedication can be given, if prescribed.

Patients are usually accompanied to the theatre by a ward nurse and information handed over to the anaesthetic nurse, assistant or anaesthetist in the anaesthetic room. The ward nurse should stay with the patient until they have been cannulated (if required) and they are anaesthetised.

Patients being prepared for theatre will require the following equipment:

- identification bracelets,
- allergy bands (if used in your area),
- theatre gown,
- anti-embolic stockings,
- labelled containers for dentures, glasses and/or hearing aid (if required),
- hypoallergenic tape (to cover wedding bands/rings),
- nail varnish remover (if nail varnish is worn),
- patient's records/documentation including medical records, consent form, drug chart, fluid chart,

medication chart (e.g. insulin, etc.), ECG recordings (if performed), X-ray films, scans, blood test results, anaesthetic assessment, record and pre-operative checklist.

Most patients may feel anxious and vulnerable while being prepared for their operation, so it is important to allow the patient to express any concerns they may have and to invite questions.

FASTING: ADULTS AND CHILDREN

It is important to read your local policies and pre-operative protocols in your area. The final decision about the timing and the type of fluid rests with the anaesthetist responsible for the care of the patient.

Royal College of Nursing (2005) recommendations suggest the following.

Adults

Use the '2 and 6 rule':

- 2: intake of water up to 2 hours before induction of anaesthesia,
- 6: a minimum pre-operative fasting time of 6 hours for food (solids, milk and milk-containing drinks).

The anaesthetic team should consider further interventions for patients at higher risk of regurgitation and aspiration.

Resumption of oral intake in healthy adults should be encouraged as soon as the patient is ready, providing there are no contraindications.

Children

Use the '2, 4 and 6 rule':

- 2: intake of water and other clear fluid up to 2 hours before induction of anaesthesia,
- 4: breast milk up to 4 hours before,
- 6: formula milk, cow's milk or solids up to 6 hours before.

The anaesthetic team should consider further interventions for children at higher risk of regurgitation and aspiration.

Resumption of oral fluids can be offered to healthy children when they are fully awake following anaesthesia, providing there are no contraindications.

MANAGEMENT OF MEDICATIONS

Unless otherwise stated, all prescribed medication should be given on the day of surgery, with a maximum of 60 mL of water during the fasting period. You will need to check your local protocol but Table 8.1 shows guidelines for the management of certain medications for elective surgery according to one NHS trust.

Table 8.1 Guidelines for the management of medication for elective surgery of certain medications

Medication	Major surgery	Minor surgery	Restart
Anticoagulant: aspirin	Continue*	Continue*	Next day
Anticoagulant: dipyridamole	Stop 24 hours pre-op*	Stop 24 hours pre-op*	Next day
Cardiac: β-blockers	Continue	Continue	
Cardiac: α-blockers	Omit morning of surgery and for 48 hours post-op	Omit morning of surgery	When blood pressure stable
Cardiac: diuretics	Continue	Continue	
Cardiac: statins	Continue	Continue	
Respiratory: inhalers/ nebulisers	Continue	Continue	
Endocrine: metformin	Omit 12 hours before surgery	Omit 12 hours before surgery	When eating and drinking
Endocrine: insulin	Omit on morning of surgery; may require a sliding scale	Omit on morning; patient first on list	Will have separate guideline
Endocrine: hormone-replacement therapy	Stop 6 weeks pre-op	Continue	When fully mobile for 2 weeks

(continued)

Table 8.1 *(Continued)*

Medication	Major surgery	Minor surgery	Restart
Endocrine: progesterone-only pill	Continue	Continue	
Endocrine: steroids	Continue	Continue	
Endocrine: tamoxifen	Stop 4 weeks pre-op	Continue	When mobile
Neurology: lithium	Stop 24 hours pre-op	Continue	As soon as possible once urea and electrolytes blood test is normal
Neurology: antiepileptics	Continue	Continue	
Neurology: antiparkinsons	Continue	Continue	
Analgesics: morphine sulphate tablets/opiates	Continue	Continue	
Analgesics: NSAIDs	Continue	Continue	
Gastrointestinal: ranitidine	Continue	Continue	

*Aspirin/dipyridamole may be stopped if for primary prevention only (asymptomatic patients). Patients who have had a myocardial infarction, angina, coronary stents, stroke, transient ischemic attack (often called a mini stroke, or temporary loss of blood flow to part of the brain) or peripheral vascular disease should stay on aspirin or dipyridamole in the peri-operative period, if taking both drugs.

NSAID, non-steroidal anti-inflammatory drug.

Adapted with permission to reproduce granted by North Bristol NHS Trust and University Hospitals Bristol NHS Foundation Trust.

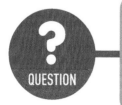

Question 8.3 Patients undergoing major surgery who require insulin need to have this drug omitted on the morning of surgery. It then states that they may require a 'sliding scale'. What is meant by a sliding scale?

INTRA-OPERATIVE CARE

Intra-operative care relates to the physical and psychological care given to a patient in the anaesthetic room and theatre until they are transferred to the recovery room, when their post-operative care starts. In this care environment you will come across circulating nurses, scrub nurses and operating department practitioners (or ODPs). It is their duty to anticipate and meet the needs of the surgeon and patient.

A scrub nurse has the responsibility to be 'scrubbed in' to ensure that a sterile technique is used throughout the surgical procedure to reduce the risk of contamination. The scrub nurse also hands surgical tools and other equipment to the surgeon. And, as in the movies, it is also their responsibility to dab sweat from the surgeon's forehead and meet any other of the surgeon's needs during the procedure. The scrub nurse also reports to the doctor if the patient's vital signs become a cause of concern.

A circulating nurse is the go-between for the operating room and the hospital, and is generally not scrubbed in. The initial assessment of the patient is conducted by the circulating nurse as they enter the anaesthetic room. The circulating nurse also assists the surgeon and scrub nurse as they clean and prepare for surgery. They may also be required to hand packages and supplies to the scrub nurse and may also be expected to pass messages to other staff members or the patient's family. The circulating nurse counts opened packages and all supplies used to ensure that nothing untoward has been left inside the patient, such as swabs. Many of the scrub and circulating nurses' duties are shared in order for the operating theatre to run smoothly.

POST-OPERATIVE CARE

After surgery the patient is transferred to the recovery room. The post-operative care process begins with the critical care post-anaesthetic recovery period and ends with the patient being discharged to a high-dependency area, hospital ward or home; all depending on the surgery and clinical state of the patient. This is usually conducted once the patient is stable, conscious and orientated.

Vital signs, wound care assessment and pain management are nursing care activities performed in the post-operative period. The post-operative care continues until the patient is discharged from the hospital setting and beyond (it may include suture removal by a practice nurse and receiving physiotherapy as an out-patient, for example).

TEST YOUR KNOWLEDGE

1 What are the three phases of the surgical procedure?
2 Name three categories of anaesthesia.
3 Name the cyclical stages of the nursing process.
4 What is the '2, 4 and 6 rule' for children fasting before an operation, according to the Royal College of Nursing's guidelines?
5 According to one NHS trust's medicine protocol (that of the North Bristol NHS Trust), how long should the drug lithium be stopped prior to major surgery?
6 What, or who, is an ODP?

KEY POINTS

- The meaning of peri-operative care.
- The pre-admission assessment.
- The nursing assessment and the nursing process.
- Pre-operative preparation.
- Fasting protocols for adults and children.
- Management of medications.
- Post-operative care.

Bibliography

Aitkenhead, A., Rowbotham, D. and Smith, G. (2001) *Textbook of Anaesthesia*. Churchill Livingstone, London.

Association of Anaesthetists of Great Britain and Ireland (2010) *Pre-operative Assessment and Patient Preparation: The Role of the Anaesthetist*. Association of Anaesthetists of Great Britain and Ireland, London.

Department of Health (2009) *Reference Guide to Consent for Examination or Treatment*. Department of Health, London.

House of Commons Health Committee (2005) *The Prevention of Venous Thromboembolism in Hospitalised Patients: Second Report of the Session 2004–2005*. House of Commons Health Committee, Stationery Office, London.

Layzell, M. (2008) Current interventions and approaches to postoperative pain management. *British Journal of Nursing* 17(7), 414–419.

National Institute for Health and Clinical Excellence (2010) *Venous Thromboembolism: Reducing the Risk of Venous Thromboembolism (Deep Vein Thrombosis and Pulmonary Embolism in Patients Admitted to Hospital)*. National Institute for Health and Clinical Excellence, London.

National Patient Safety Agency (2010) *Checking Pregnancy Before Surgery: Rapid Response Report*. NPSA/2010/RRR011. National Patient Safety Agency, London.

North Bristol NHS Trust (2011) *Pre-operative Fasting in Adults Guidelines*. Policy number CP7e. North Bristol NHS Trust, Bristol.

Oshodi, T. (2004) Clinical skills: an evidence-based approach to preoperative fasting. *British Journal of Nursing* 13(16), 958–962.

Pudner, R. (ed.) (2005) *Nursing the Surgical Patient*, 2nd edn. Bailliere Tindall, London.

Royal College of Nursing (2005) *Perioperative Fasting in Adults and Children – an RCN Guideline for the Multidisciplinary Team*. Royal College of Nursing, London.

Walker, L. and Lamont, S. (2007) Use and application of graduated elastic compression stockings. *Nursing Standard* 21(42), 41–45.

Wicker, P. and O'Neill, J. (2006) *Caring for the Peri-operative Patient*. Blackwell Publishing, Oxford.

Chapter 9

ANAPHYLAXIS

Care Skills for Nurses, First Edition. Claire Boyd
© 2014 John Wiley & Sons, Ltd. Published 2014 by John Wiley & Sons, Ltd.

LEARNING OUTCOMES

By the end of this chapter you will have an understanding of the theory and practice of managing an anaphylactic episode.

Allergic reactions (Figure 9.1) are caused by substances in the environment, known as allergens. Most commonly these are pollen from trees and grasses, house dust mites, wasp and bee stings and certain foodstuffs, such as peanuts, milk and eggs. Asthma and skin disorders can also be allergy-related.

One third of the UK population is now estimated to have an allergy, the most common one being caused by pollen from trees and grasses. Most allergic reactions can occur within minutes of exposure to the allergen, but some can present with a slower onset.

The UK Science and Technology Committee (a House of Lords committee) found that there has been a rapid growth in the number of people suffering from allergies, as a result of both genetic and environmental factors. The phenomenon has been described as an epidemic, costing the NHS over £1 billon per year to treat (BBC 2007). Milder allergic reactions, where there is no deterioration in cardiovascular or respiratory function, and which are not life-threatening, may not require any treatment.

Anaphylaxis is the most severe form of allergic reaction and is life-threatening because it does involve the airway, breathing and circulation, and can be triggered by a very broad range of agents. Each year over 6000 people in

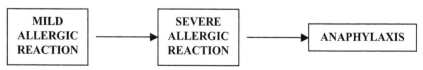

Figure 9.1 Types of allergic reaction

England are admitted to hospital because of an allergy; a quarter of these people have anaphylaxis that is severe enough to be potentially life-threatening due to the involvement of the airways, causing breathing difficulties. People can die from anaphylaxis if treatment is not obtained quickly enough, as they go into anaphylactic shock (this is when the airway, breathing and circulation are involved). They may have presented initially with just a 'lump in the throat', tingling in the mouth or a rash. The UK Resuscitation Council reports an average of 20 deaths per year as a result of anaphylaxis.

As a health carer you will be involved in drug administration, and we do not want those in our care to suffer an adverse reaction due to something that we have administered, be it food or medication. It is possible to aspirate the stomach contents by gastric lavage if a patient is given a drug to which they subsequently react, or to remove medication that has been administered rectally or vaginally; all to minimise the exposure to the drug. When administering drugs by the intravenous route we need to know about anaphylaxis and how to manage an adverse event. This is because intravenous drugs enter the body system quickly and there is no recall once the drug has been administered (although there is often an antidote).

WHAT IS ANAPHYLAXIS?

Anaphylaxis is likely when all of the following three criteria are met:

1 life-threatening and/or breathing and/or circulation problems,
2 skin and/or mucosal changes,
3 sudden onset and rapid progression of symptoms.

The Nomenclature Review Committee of the World Allergy Organization (Johansson et al. 2003) give the following definition of anaphylaxis:

> Anaphylaxis is a severe, life-threatening, and generalised or systemic hypersensitivity reaction.

In other words, anaphylaxis is an exaggerated response of a previous sensitised individual to a foreign antigenic material. Therefore the individual will need to have had previous exposure to the substance (the antigen; see below for a discussion about allergens and antigens). However, there may be no knowledge by the individual of this previous exposure if the adverse effects were mild.

Phylaxis is a word seldom used in health care, but means 'protection' in Greek. So what do you think *anaphylaxis* means? It has the opposite meaning: 'without protection'.

WHAT IS AN ANAPHYLACTOID EVENT?

An anaphylactoid event occurs on first exposure to an antigen, so needs no specific antibody. If someone collapses, there is no need to stand over them and wonder 'Hmm! I wonder if this is an anaphylactic or an anaphylactoid event?' Both present with the same symptoms and require the same treatment. Both can be fatal. Subsequent events will be anaphylactic, as following the first event antibodies will be made by the body. The antibodies will be triggered by exposure to the same antigen in the future.

This was misunderstood and for many years medics only gave the first intravenous antibiotic injections to patients, and nurses could only give the second or third doses. We now know that a reaction to an antibiotic is more likely to occur on the second dose onwards, when antibodies in the body recognise the antigen from last time and start an immune reaction.

Sometimes, individuals experience very mild symptoms on first exposure and do not recognise this as a reaction to a new drug or something they have just eaten.

WHAT'S THE DIFFERENCE BETWEEN AN ANTIBODY AND AN ANTIGEN?

An antibody is a protein produced by the immune system in response to the presence of an antigen, a protein that is in or on material that the body 'sees' as 'foreign'. An allergen is an antigen that causes an allergic reaction. The body attacks this 'enemy' material – the antigen – by producing antibodies. In an allergic reaction this sets off a cascade of chemicals, such as histamines and cortisone, creating the symptoms of a severe reaction.

Such a reaction can affect the airway, breathing and circulation, resulting in the symptoms of **laryngeal oedema** (or swelling), **bronchospasm** and **hypotension**. As the throat is very vascular, swelling to this area may be the first sign that a problem is occurring. The patient may present with a rasping/husky voice.

Unfortunately we can become allergic to anything and at any time in our lifespan. Sometimes an anaphylactic reaction can present with symptoms and signs that are very similar to life-threatening asthma: this is most common in children.

There may also be confusion between an anaphylactic reaction and a panic attack. Victims of previous anaphylaxis can be prone to panic attacks if they think they have been re-exposed to the allergen that caused the previous problem. Other non-life-threatening conditions are:

- fainting (vasovagal episode),
- panic attack,
- breath-holding in children,
- idiopathic (non-allergic) urticaria or angio-oedema.

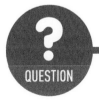
QUESTION

Question 9.1 Unravel the words to find the four most common trigger groups for an anaphylaxis event.

1 DOSOF
2 DETINCEJ MNOVE
3 GSRUD
4 TELAX

FOODS

In children, foods are the most common trigger for a severe allergic reaction:

- peanuts (about 1 in 200 people are allergic to them),
- tree nuts: walnuts, pecans, pistachios, cob nuts, cashews, almonds, etc.,
- shellfish,
- fish,
- milk,
- pulses: lentils,
- sesame,
- soy,
- wheat,
- eggs,
- some fruit and vegetables.

Many foodstuffs, and other products, contain a problematic antigen that may not be obvious in the actual item. For instance, the main ingredient of some cardiac drugs is based on avocado and people with diary intolerance need to ensure that the outer casings of tablets do not contain milk proteins, which are commonly used in antibiotics.

Also, many breads or biscuits contain peanuts, or are produced in factories where peanut-based foods are also prepared, contaminating other non-peanut-based foodstuffs. A shampoo often used to treat cradle cap contains peanuts: arachis oil. What a minefield! Thankfully, European regulations now require ingredients to be listed on food packaging.

INJECTED VENOM

Some of the known injected-venom triggers are:

- bees,
- wasps,
- yellow jackets,
- hornets,
- ants.

Why, do you think, is snake or spider venom not on the list? After all, many people like to keep exotic snakes and spiders from overseas. Well, I posed this question to a specialist and was informed that it is because it takes approximately 5 minutes to die of respiratory arrest following a potent spider or snake bite, which is not long enough for the cascade of chemicals to be released to cause an anaphylaxis event. In other words, the venom will kill you before the anaphylaxis will!

DRUGS

Medications are the most common trigger for anaphylaxis in adults. You may have seen television medical dramas in which someone undergoing an operation is asked by the anaesthetist, as they are slowly injecting the anaesthetic, 'any metallic taste in your mouth?' Or perhaps you have been asked this question while 'going under'. Do you know why? It is because a metallic taste in the mouth is often the first indication that someone is starting to react to a medication. Some other known drug triggers are:

- penicillin and cephalosporin antibiotics,
- aspirin and non-steroidal anti-inflammatory drugs,
- sulpha antibiotics,
- allopurinol,
- muscle relaxants,
- vaccines,
- radio-contrast media,
- anti-hypertensives,
- insulin,
- blood products.

QUESTION

Question 9.2   Can you explain what the following drugs are for?

- Cephalosporin antibiotics
- Sulpha antibiotics
- Allopurinol

LATEX

We know that latex is all around us in nature. For instance, dandelion 'milk' contains latex. But the problematic substance is that from the rubber tree. In health care exposure to this material commonly occurs via gloves. It has been estimated that less than 1% of the population are allergic to latex, but the problem is more prevalent among those working in health care and in the hairdressing industry. We also know that certain groups of individuals have an increased risk of sensitivity, such as people who have had multiple surgical procedures (due to latex proteins entering the body from the surgeon's gloves), and those who suffer from dermatitis, asthma or food allergies.

Patients who state on admission to hospital that they are allergic to certain fruits (the top three being bananas, avocado and kiwi fruits) must be treated as latex-sensitive. Why? It is because these fruits contain similar protein chains to those found in latex. Therefore, we must not expose them to this protein. Many NHS trusts do not allow latex gloves in the workplace, except for 'high-risk' procedures and in surgery during operations.

Foodstuffs and plants that contain similar protein chains to latex are:

- apples,
- **avocados**,
- **bananas**,
- celery,
- cherries,
- chestnuts,
- *Ficus* (trees of the fig family),
- figs,
- grapes,
- **kiwi fruits**,
- mangoes,
- melons,
- passion fruit,
- peaches,
- pears,

- pistachios,
- potatoes,
- ragweed,
- strawberries,
- tomatoes.

ROUTES

Anaphylaxis not only occurs with medication being administered via the intravenous route, although this is a very quick mode of entry. Any of the bodily routes can cause a reaction to occur, because the allergen has entered the body, such as:

- oral,
- rectal,
- vaginal,
- inhaled,
- subcutaneous,
- intravenous,
- topical.

WHAT ARE THE SIGNS AND SYMPTOMS OF ANAPHYLAXIS?

Although we have discussed how a true anaphylactic event has airway, breathing and circulatory involvement, anaphylaxis can be broken up into five areas of response:

- cutaneous,
- respiratory,
- central nervous system,
- gastrointestinal,
- cardiovascular.

Cutaneous

This pertains to the skin. An individual may have a reaction to something that causes skin involvement: this may or may not go on to cause an anaphylactic reaction, and so it should be treated promptly. Cutaneous involvement may present as:

- swelling (angio-oedema),
- urticaria (hives),
- redness (erythema),
- itching (pruritus),
- sweating.

Angio-oedema may cause occlusion of the airway. The urticaria can be painful as well as unsightly, as may erythema. Pruritus may present as a maddening itch, which can occur when an individual is having a reaction to penicillin. Chlorphenamine meleate, more commonly known by its trade name Piriton, may be prescribed in this case to relieve the irritation. Reassuringly, most patients who have skin changes caused by allergy do not go on to develop an anaphylactic reaction.

Respiratory

Respiratory involvement may start off as a 'lump in the throat'. This is due to laryngeal oedema as the airways are starting to close over. Other respiratory involvement may include:

- wheezing,
- dyspnoea, with increased respiratory rate,
- rhinitis,
- laryngeal obstruction leading to stridor,
- hypoxia,
- respiratory arrest.

Any difficulty breathing is life-threatening. Oxygen should be administered and the airway cleared, with an laryngeal adjunct, if necessary. But the most important thing is to *call for help*.

Central Nervous System

A patient may first experience a feeling of faintness and/or dizziness due to a lowering of blood pressure: hypotension. Other signs may be:

- confusion (due to hypoxia),
- feeling of impending doom,

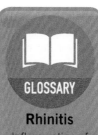

GLOSSARY

Rhinitis
Inflammation of the membranes lining the nose, causing extreme running of secretions or sometimes blockage. Antihistamines may relieve the symptoms.

Stridor
High-pitched noise heard on inspiration, caused by upper airway obstruction. This is a medical emergency.

- apprehension/anxiety,
- metallic taste in the mouth,
- altered level of consciousness.

Initially it may be difficult to distinguish whether a patient is confused by being in hospital and losing their bearings, or whether the confusion is the start of a reaction to a drug that has not long been administered, causing decreased oxygen brain perfusion. The 'feeling of impending doom' is a strange one, as this indicates central nervous system involvement. I have only ever seen this once in my nursing career, whereby a patient asked me tell his wife that she was 'a wonderful woman' before he collapsed!

Gastrointestinal

Depending on an individual's trigger, injected drugs can have a quicker reaction than injected venom (stings), which in turn have a quicker reaction than orally ingested triggers. Gastrointestinal symptoms may not be immediately life-threatening (but in very small children and the elderly this *will* be more critical).

Cardiovascular

Remember that true anaphylaxis involves the airway, breathing and circulation. Initially a patient may present with signs of shock, becoming pale and clammy, and feeling faint and dizzy. Other signs of cardiovascular symptoms are:

- hypotension,
- tachycardia,
- cardiac arrhythmias,
- cardiac arrest.

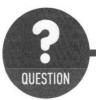
QUESTION

Question 9.3 Would you sit someone up whom you suspected of having an anaphylaxis event?

MANAGEMENT

Prevention is always better than cure, so the best prevention is not to expose our patients to a known allergen! It is important that we know our patients well, by making a good assessment on admission, if in hospital, and checking our patient's history of adverse reactions before prescribing or administering any medication. After any new treatment, patients should always remain in the location for at least 10 minutes so that we can observe for any adverse reactions. Medical treatment can be given immediately in this situation, if required. How many of you have been given a vaccine, perhaps for influenza or when going on holiday. Hopefully you were asked to sit down and observed for this amount of time. Anyone experiencing a reaction should be laid flat, with feet raised, given oxygen (if available) and given the first line of treatment: adrenaline. As with any emergency situation, the ABCDE assessment will be performed:

A   Airway,
B   Breathing,
C   Circulation,
D   Disability,
E   Exposure.

Patients could have either an A, B or C problem or any combination. Table 9.1 shows how the ABCDE assessment relates to an anaphylactic event.

Table 9.1 ABCDE assessment and anaphylaxis

Assessement	Symptoms
A	Airway swelling, e.g. throat and tongue swelling (pharyngeal/laryngeal oedema). The patient has difficulty breathing and swallowing and feels that the throat is closing up.
B	See Respiratory section under What are the signs and symptoms of anaphylaxis?
C	See Cardiovascular section under What are the signs and symptoms of anaphylaxis?

Assessement	Symptoms
D	Airway, breathing and circulation problems also alter the patient's neurological status due to decreased brain perfusion. The patient's blood glucose should be obtained to rule out hypoglycaemia and the prescription chart should also be checked. See Central nervous system section under What are the signs and symptoms of anaphylaxis?
E	Fully expose the body and examine the patient thoroughly. Remember to minimise heat loss and to maintain the patient's dignity. Don't forget to call for help. See Cutaneous section under What are the signs and symptoms of anaphylaxis?

It is important to remember that a patient should receive immediate medical treatment when experiencing symptoms indicative of anaphylaxis. The flowchart in Figure 9.2 shows healthcare management of an anaphylactic event.

ADRENALINE

In the hospital environment, adrenaline (epinephrine) is located on the resuscitation trolley in the 'first-line' emergency drug box. Nurses working in the community should have easy access to their supplies of adrenaline. **Adrenaline for anaphylaxis is expressed as 1:1000**, which means that there is 1 mg of the drug in every 1 mL of fluid (1 g in 1000 mL). In an emergency, nurses can administer 0.5 mL (0.5 mg, or 500 µg) intramuscularly, usually in the more assessable mid outer thigh: the vastus lateralis muscle. As time is of the essence it may not be appropriate to remove outer clothes, such as tights and/or trousers. Five minutes later a second injection of 0.5 mL/0.5 mg can be given. Some adrenaline comes ready prepared in the syringe; in some areas you may have to draw it up yourself. It is important not to get confused with adrenaline administered for cardiopulmonary resuscitation: this is expressed as 1:10 000, which means 1 mg in every 10 mL. Although this is a larger volume (1 g in 10 000 mL) it is more potent as it is given intravenously.

In many clinical areas staff can only administer adrenaline when key factors are in place: they must

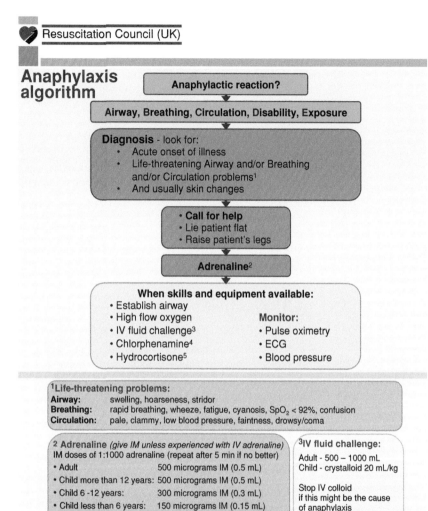

Figure 9.2 Treatment for an anaphylactic event. Permission to reproduce this image is granted by The Resuscitation Council (UK).

have attended an intravenous study day, be up to date with their basic life support training, have attended anaphylaxis training, have a PGD in place and been assessed as competent.

What is a PGD?

PGD stands for Patient Group Directive, whereby nurses are able to administer medicines such as adrenaline using a group protocol arrangement that has been signed by a doctor, pharmacist or other responsible people or person (named healthcare professionals). So, a trained nurse may be able to administer the adrenaline and can ask a colleague to prepare the 'second line' of drugs, which need to be prescribed. These may include antihistamines, nebulisers, hydrocortisones, oxygen, etc.

Adrenaline needs to be stored at room temperature, protected from direct light. Always check the expiry date, as adrenaline does have a very short shelf life.

Patients who know that they have a sensitivity carry their own adrenaline syringe, known as an Epipen. They usually only contain 0.3 mg (300 micrograms), not the 0.5 mg (500 micrograms) we give in hospital. Children's own adrenaline depends on their age, but a pen may only contain 0.15 mg (150 micrograms) of the drug.

Cautions for administering adrenaline are as follows, although the decision to treat may not change in an emergency situation:

- hyperthyroidism,
- diabetes mellitus,
- heart disease,
- hypertension,
- phaeochromocytoma,
- arrhythmias,
- pregnancy,
- cerebrovascular disease,
- cerebral arteriosclerosis,
- narrow-angle glaucoma.

GLOSSARY

Phaeochromocytoma
Tumour of the adrenal glands. Symptoms may include headache, sweating, hypertension and palpitations.

How Does Adrenaline Work?

Now for the scientific bit! During anaphylaxis, the blood vessels leak, bronchial tissues swell and the blood pressure drops, causing the choking and collapse.

Adrenaline acts quickly to:

- constrict the blood vessels,
- relax the smooth muscles in the lungs to improve breathing,
- stimulate the heart's contractility,
- help stop swelling around the face and lips (the angio-oedema).

AFTERCARE

After an episode of anaphylaxis the patient will need reassurance, rest and continued observation. The patient will also need to receive health education about why this episode happened and be advised to avoid the trigger, if possible, in the future. Many patients like to carry a patient information in the form of a medical alert bracelet in case they are unable to communicate verbally at the time of an attack. Healthcare professionals may also complete a yellow card, found in the *British National Formulary*, to alert the Department of Health that a particular drug has caused an adverse reaction. Patients can also carry Life Line cards, again to alert others of their condition during an anaphylactic event.

BIPHASIC RESPONSE

This is known as a 'rebound', whereby the symptoms may return in some people after the initial episode and treatment. Re-occurrence can be 8–12 hours after the first attack, and patients should always be informed of this so that they can plan not to be alone. Further doses of adrenaline may be required. It is always good practice to give patients a booklet or leaflet with information for them to read in their own time, as verbal information given during their anaphylactic event may be forgotten. Remember, English may not be their first language.

DOCUMENTATION

If the incident occurred in a hospital a description of the reaction, with circumstances, timings, treatments and investigations, needs to be documented. If the incident occurred when a blood product was being administered then paperwork relating to this will need to be completed. Any suspected substance/drug/allergen should be kept while the investigation is being completed.

INVESTIGATIONS OF ANAPHYLAXIS

Clotted Blood Samples

The specific test to help confirm a diagnosis of an anaphylactic reaction is measurement of mast cell tryptase. This is taken in a blood sample obtained via venepuncture. Tryptase levels are useful in the follow-up of suspected anaphylactic reactions, not in the initial recognition and treatment. The half-life of mast cell tryptase is short (approximately 2 hours) and concentrations may be back to normal levels within 6–8 hours, so timing of any blood samples is very important.

Urine

Urine samples may also be collected immediately after the reaction and then again 2–4 hours after the incident. This is obtained to measure methylhistamine. Methylhistamine is what histamine turns into when your body inactivates it.

Immunology Therapy

Immunology therapy is when small doses of antigen are injected into patients to decrease reactions to subsequent exposures. These patients are obviously closely watched for any reactions and all tests are conducted over very strict laboratory conditions. There has been some degree of success with children exposed to peanuts.

Skin Tests

This is the only test we have to tell us what the person had a reaction too. The blood and urine sample tests for mast cell tryptase and methylhistamine just tell us that a person has *had* a reaction. Very often patients have to pay privately for these tests.

TEST YOUR KNOWLEDGE

1 What is the main generating trigger for an anaphylactic event in children?
2 What is the main generating trigger for an anaphylactic event in adults?
3 What is angio-oedema?
4 What is urticaria?
5 How does adrenaline work?
6 Name some of the known food triggers for anaphylaxis.

KEY POINTS

- Definition of anaphylaxis.
- Common triggers for an allergic reaction.
- Signs and symptoms of an anaphylactic event.
- Management of anaphylaxis.
- How adrenaline works.
- Aftercare and documentation.

Bibliography

BBC (2007) Allergy epidemic gets 'poor care'. http://news.bbc.co.uk/1/hi/health/7012794.stm.

British National Formulary (2010) *British National Formulary No 59*. British Medical Association and Royal Pharmaceutical Society of Great Britain, London.

Henderson, N. (1998) Anaphylaxis. *Nursing Standard* 12(47), 49–55.

Johansson, S.G., Bieber, T., Dahl, R., Friedmann, P.S., Lanier, B.Q. et al. (2004) Revised nomenclature for allergy for global use: Report of the Nomenclature Review Committee of the World Allergy Organization, October 2003. *Journal of Allergy and Clinical Immunology* 113(5), 832–836.

Hughes, G. and Fitzharris, P. (1999) Managing acute anaphylaxis. *British Medical Journal*, 319, 1–2.

Krause, R.S. (2006) *Anaphylaxis*. www.emedicine.com/EMERG/topic25.htm.

Linton, E. and Watson, D. (2010) Recognition, assessment and management of anaphylaxis. *Nursing Standard* 24(46), 35–39.

Resuscitation Council UK (2008) *Emergency Treatment of Anaphylactic Reactions. Guidelines for Healthcare Providers*. RCUK, London.

Royal College of Paediatrics and Child Health and the Neonatal and Paediatric Pharmacists Group (2003) *Medicines for Children*, 2nd edn. RCPCH Publications, London.

Royal College of Physicians (2009) New guidance to address soaring numbers of allergic reactions. Rcplondon.ac.uk/Archive/2009.

Website

Homepage of the Anaphylaxis Campaign: www.anaphylaxis.org.uk

Chapter 10
. . . .
ECG RECORDING

Care Skills for Nurses, First Edition. Claire Boyd
© 2014 John Wiley & Sons, Ltd. Published 2014 by John Wiley & Sons, Ltd.

LEARNING OUTCOMES

By the end of this chapter you will have an understanding of the theory and practice of performing the clinical skill of ECG recording.

An electrocardiogram, or ECG, is a diagnostic test that measures the electrical activity and muscular functions of the heart from electrodes that have been placed on the patient's chest and limbs. These electrodes transmit the electrical impulses generated by the heart to the ECG machine; the machine then produces a graph, called the ECG tracing. These results show the rate and rhythm of the heartbeat, as well as providing indirect evidence of the blood flow to the heart muscle.

Patients may ask about the possibility of getting an electrical shock from the procedure, but you can reassure them that it is not dangerous because no electricity is sent through the body. There is no risk of electrical shock, and an ECG is painless.

A standard ECG machine has 12 leads with 10 electrodes, which produce 12 electrical views of the heart (Figure 10.1). An electrode is placed on each arm and leg and the remaining six are placed across the chest wall. It is important to have training for the machine in use in your area.

HEART MONITORS

A heart monitor may be used and requires only three electrode leads. Their tabs are placed as follows: one on the right shoulder (this is the **negative** electrode), one placed on the left shoulder (the **earth** electrode) and one placed on the lower left abdomen (the **positive** electrode). These monitors only measure the rate and rhythm of the heartbeat. Therefore, this monitoring does not constitute a complete ECG. The electrodes are usually colour-coded, so

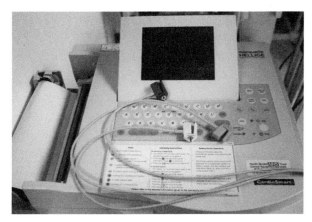

Figure 10.1 An ECG machine.

you will need to familiarise yourself with the instructions for each particular machine and set of electrodes, as different machines and leads use different colour-coded tabs. Note that five-lead monitors may also be in use in many clinical areas.

Patients may require continuous cardiac monitoring due to:

- chest pain,
- post-myocardial infarction,
- arrhythmias or potential arrhythmias,
- starting a newly prescribed drug treatment,
- having taken an overdose,
- having abnormally low or high blood chemistry.

BASIC ANATOMY OF THE HEART

The heart has four chambers: the right and left atrium and the right and left ventricle. It is the right side of the heart that collects blood from the body and pumps it to the lungs, whereas the left side of the heart receives the blood from the lungs and pumps it to the body. Like all muscles and cells the heart requires oxygen and nutrients to function; these are supplied by arteries that originate from the aorta.

The heart contains specialised cells that initiate and conduct electrical impulses. This conduction system comprises:

- sinus node (sinoatrial or SA node),
- atrioventricular node (AV node),
- bundle of His,
- bundle branches (right and left),
- Purkinje fibres.

Electrically the heart can be divided into upper and lower chambers: the heartbeat *originates* in the SA node. This SA node acts independently of the brain to generate electricity for the heart to beat and is often referred to as the automatic pacemaker. The rate at which the SA node fires is dependent on the vagus nerve: an increase in vagal activity *slows* the heart rate and a decrease in vagal activity *speeds up* the heart rate. Atropine is used to block the vagus nerve when we need to increase the heart rate.

The SA node fires and the electrical impulse spreads across the atria causing atrial contraction: the **P wave**. This electrical impulse stimulates the atria to squeeze and push blood into the ventricles of the heart (known as myocardial contractions). As this is happening, the impulse is slowed down, presenting as a straight line (isoelectric line) between the end of the P wave and the beginning of the QRS complex.

The electrical impulse progresses to the AV node down to the bundle of His and then through the right and left bundle branches and ending in the Purkinje fibres, which stimulates the ventricles to contract to pump blood to the body and lungs. The septum (dividing wall) is depolarised from left to right with the left ventricle exerting more influence than the right. This ventricular depolarisation and contraction produces the **QRS complex**. The ventricles then repolarise: this is the **T wave**.

Figure 10.2 shows how the P wave, QRS complex and T wave present on an ECG recording.

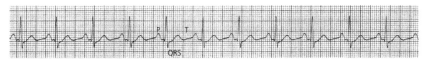

Figure 10.2 The ECG and its relation to cardiac contraction (Jevon 2010).

THE PROCEDURE

Before the ECG can be recorded there are various items of equipment that need to be gathered:

- the ECG machine,
- disposable razor,
- tissues,
- alcohol wipes,
- 10 disposable pre-gelled electrodes (check expiry date, as dry gel inhibits conduction),
- gloves (if there is any possibility of contamination with blood or other bodily fluids).

Pull the curtains around the bed space for privacy and dignity and gain consent. Patients will then be asked to remove upper clothing and lie semi-recumbent.

Females will need to remove their bras. Some patients may require assistance to undress. Some patients will be unable to lie semi-recumbent or flat so may need to sit in a chair for this procedure. In this case the patient should not sit higher than 45 degrees and this should be recorded on the tracing. It is important to keep the patient warm to reduce muscle tremor (shivering). Explain the procedure to the patient, keeping them well informed.

PERFORMING THE ECG

1 Wash your hands before and after the procedure.
2 Unless it is an emergency situation, consent will need to be gained before the procedure can start.
3 Ensure the bed is at a comfortable height for performing the procedure.
4 Once you are sure the patient is comfortable, informed and warm, the ECG recording can proceed.

5   To ensure good contact, if the skin is greasy, wipe the skin with a 70% isopropyl alcohol swab and then dry the area with clean gauze. If you place the electrode on wet alcohol it will adversely affect the trace. Place the pre-gelled electrode over the swabbed area. If the skin is not greasy you can apply the pre-gelled electrode directly to the skin.

6   If the patient has excess chest hair it may need removing. Most pre-gelled tabs do stick to the skin despite the hairs; you will have to use your own judgement, or if you are not sure ask a more experienced member of staff for advice. If clipping is required (shaving is not recommended for infection-control reasons) the patient may feel more comfortable clipping himself. If you have to clip the patient, be careful if the patient has any skin blemishes or spots, and be vigilant when clipping around the nipple area. Also, if necessary, take into consideration the patient's cultural background; gain permission and consent before clipping either chest or limb hair.

7   If the skin is wet, dry the area before applying the electrode.

8   It is important to remember that correct lead placement is essential and the tabs should be placed in the same (correct) place for each individual recording. If the patient has abnormal anatomy, i.e. kyphoscoliosis, then you should still follow the same principles, using the ribs as guides, as the trace can be replicated when necessary.

9   If the patient has eczema, psoriasis or other skin conditions that may prevent correct lead placement, place the tabs as close to the correct area as possible, record the trace and document clearly why there was abnormal lead placement.

10   If you are recording a trace on a patient with large breasts then the general rule is to make an assessment as to the easiest access to the rib spaces. If access is easiest by placing the tabs under the breast, that is fine, or if access to the rib space is easiest on top of the breast, then is fine as well. You will have to make your own assessment and use your own judgement.

PLACEMENT OF THE LEADS

The leads should be placed in the following positions, which you will need to familiarise yourself with during your training in this clinical procedure.

Chest Leads

C1: fourth intercostal space, right sternal border
C2: fourth intercostal space, left sternal border
C3: midway between V2 and V4
C4: fifth intercostal space, left midclavicular line
C5: fifth intercostal space, left anterior axillary line
C6: fifth intercostal space, left midaxillary line

Limb Leads

Limb leads are often colour-coded; the colours used may vary by manufacturer, so do check. But each lead can be identified by the following abbreviations:

R: right arm
L: left arm
F: left leg
N: right leg

RECORDING

Once the electrodes have been attached to the patient and before the recording is obtained, and in order to get a good trace, the following needs to be addressed:

- ask patient to relax,
- ask patient to put both arms by their side,
- ask patient to breath gently,
- ask patient not to talk during the trace,
- ensure the leads are tangle-free and not crossed.

You will have to establish whether the machine is calibrated correctly (this can be done by following the manufacturer's instructions). Calibration is usually confirmed by the presence of the calibration 'spike' recorded on the ECG; different machines may vary in the size and shape of the calibration spike, so it is important to check with your individual machine.

AFTERCARE

Once the recording has been completed the patient may need help removing the electrodes. Take care when removing them: if the patient has fragile skin the removal of the electrode may cause trauma, so remove them carefully. Also, check for signs of an allergic reaction. If allergic signs are present (redness, itchiness, soreness directly relating to electrode placement areas), inform the doctor and the patient. Record what you have seen.

If clinically indicated (e.g. acute chest pain or arrhythmia) the ECG tabs may need to stay in place (for serial recordings); if so, be careful when unhooking the leads from the tabs, trying not to disturb them.

The patient may become anxious following the procedure and may ask you what the ECG shows. Take care when answering; remember you are only *recording* and not *interpreting* the ECG, which is an advanced clinical skill.

Help the patient to re-dress, if needed.

NOTE: not all ECGs are performed in a routine manner; ECGs are often needed in response to an emergency situation. Despite the urgency, the above principles must be adhered to. If a person is suffering from a cardiac-related condition the correct recording of the ECG is essential for helping the assessment and treatment of the patient.

DOCUMENTATION

Inform nursing and medical staff *immediately that the recording has been obtained*. If the machine does not record the patient's name automatically you will need to write the following on the tracing:

* the patient's name,
* the patient's date of birth,

- date of ECG,
- time of ECG,
- whether the filter setting was on or off,
- the intensity of any chest pain that the patient is experiencing.

PROBLEMS WITH THE RECORDING

Problems may be encountered with an ECG recoding, some of which are outlined in Table 10.1.

Table 10.1 Problems that may be encountered with an ECG recording

Problem	Possible remedy
Straight line	Check the patient, then check the C2 lead. Asystole rarely produces a straight line.
Poor-quality ECG	Check all the connections and brightness display. Check all electrodes are correctly attached. Ensure the skin where the electrodes are placed is dry; wipe the skin with an alcohol swab if necessary.
Interference and artefacts	The causes may be poor electrode contact, patient movement and interference (possibly caused by infusion pumps). Apply electrodes over bone to remedy.
Wandering baseline	Usually caused by patient movement. Reposition electrodes away from the lower ribs.
Small ECG complexes	Could be caused by pericardial effusion, obesity and hypothyroidism. Could be a technical problem: check the correct ECG monitoring leads have been selected.
Incorrect heart rate display	Results in small QRS complexes on the paper trace, possibly due to interference and muscle movement. Keep the patient warm.

WHAT DOES IT ALL MEAN?

Normal ECG results will show:

Heart rate = 60–100 beats per minute
Heart rhythm = consistent and even

Possible abnormal results are shown in Table 10.2.

Table 10.2 Abnormal ECG recordings

Problem	Possible cause
Abnormal heart rhythms (arrhythmias)	Heart valve disease
Cardiac muscle defect	Inflammation of the heart (myocarditis)
Congenital heart defect	Changes in the amount of electrolytes (chemicals in the blood)
Coronary artery disease	Past heart attack
Ectopic heartbeat	Present or impending heart attack
Enlargement of the heart	Slower-than-normal heart rate (bradycardia)
Faster-than-normal heart rate (tachycardia)	Interference on machine, i.e. 'electrical noise'

A NORMAL ECG

This chapter has looked at how to record an ECG. Interpreting these recordings is a separate skill. When you undertake training in ECG recording and interpretation you will be shown how to read the P and QRS complexes.

Sinus rhythm is the normal rhythm of the heart, which originates in the sinus node. This is what sinus rhythm means:

- QRS rate = 60–100 beats per minute,
- QRS rhythm = regular,
- QRS width = normal,
- P waves = present, normal,
- relationship between P waves and QRS complexes = P wave precedes each QRS complex.

Each large square (5 mm) on the ECG readout represents 0.2 seconds; therefore, there are five large squares to a second and 300 for a minute (Figure 10.3). The paper should be calibrated at 25 millimetres per second.

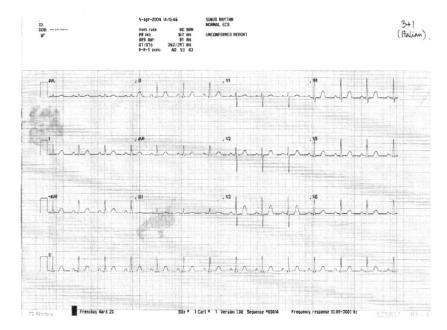

Figure 10.3 ECG paper calibration.

Sinus tachycardia means:

- QRS rate = more than 100 beats per minute,
- QRS rhythm = regular,
- QRS width = normal,
- P waves = present, normal but more than 100 beats per minute,
- relationship between P waves and QRS complexes = P wave precedes each QRS complex.

Sinus bradycardia means:

- QRS rate = less than 60 beats per minute,
- QRS rhythm = regular,
- QRS width = normal,
- P waves = present, normal but less than 60 beats per minute,
- relationship between P waves and QRS complexes = P wave precedes each QRS complex.

A Shivering Patient

Figure 10.4 shows a reading from a shivering patient.

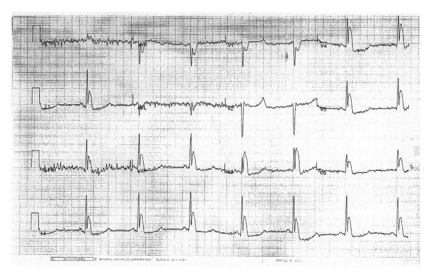

Figure 10.4 ECG tracing from shivering patient.

AC INTERFERENCE (ARTEFACT)

Figure 10.5 shows interference on the trace.

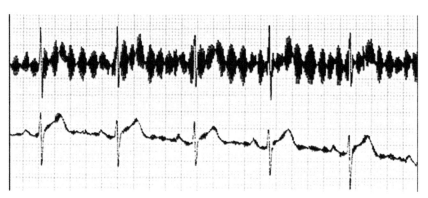

Figure 10.5 AC interference on an ECG trace.

Tricks of the Trade

As you get more experienced with ECG recordings you will be able to 'read' them, but it is good to show these simple readings to you now so that you will begin to interpret the results, to get you started.

Remember:

- keep the patient warm and relaxed,
- make sure someone sees the recording,
- correct lead placement is essential: if leads need to be placed in an 'incorrect' position then document this clearly,
- don't fall into the trap of telling the patient that 'it looks OK'.

TEST YOUR KNOWLEDGE

1 The normal recording speed of an ECG is:
   a   33 mm per second,
   b   25 mm per second,
   c   10 mm per second,
   d   60 mm per second.
2 AC interference is caused by:
   a   a low battery in the machine,
   b   the patient having a pacemaker,
   c   the patient talking during the recording,
   d   electrical interference.
3 What do you need to ask the patient to do during the ECG procedure? Pick as many as apply.
   a   Relax
   b   Not to talk during the procedure
   c   Sit upright
   d   Drink a glass of water
4 What should you say to the patient after the recording?
   a   'It looks OK.'
   b   'Oh dear, poor you!'
   c   'I need to show the recording to the medic; this is standard procedure.'
   d   'Do you want to keep the tracing?'

KEY POINTS

- The ECG machine.
- Heart monitors.
- Basic anatomy of the heart.
- Performing the ECG recording.
- Problems that may be encountered with an ECG recording.

Bibliography

Ganz, L. and Curtiss, E. (2007) Electrocardiography. In Goldman, L. and Ausiello, D. (eds), *Cecil Medicine*, 23rd edn. Saunders Elsevier, Philadelphia, PA.

Jevon, P. (2010) *Advanced Cardiac Life Support – a Guide for Nurses*, 2nd edn. Wiley Blackwell, Oxford.

Metcalfe, H. (2000) Recording a 12 lead electrocardiogram. Part 1 (Practical Procedures for Nurses. Part 40.1.2). *Nursing Times* 19, 43–44.

National Institute for Health and Clinical Excellence (2006) *Hypertension: Management of Hypertension in Adults in Primary Care*. NICE Clinical Guideline 34. National Institute for Health and Clinical Excellence, London.

National Institute for Health and Clinical Excellence (2007) *Acutely Ill Patients in Hospital: Recognition of and Response to Acute Illness in Adults in Hospital*. NICE Clinical Guideline 50. National Institute for Health and Clinical Excellence, London.

Wedro, B. (2012) *Electrocardiogram (ECG, EKG)*. www.emedicinehealth.com/electrocardiogram_ecg/article_em.htm.

Chapter 11

. . . .

NUTRITION AND HYDRATION CARE

Care Skills for Nurses, First Edition. Claire Boyd
© 2014 John Wiley & Sons, Ltd. Published 2014 by John Wiley & Sons, Ltd.

LEARNING OUTCOMES

By the end of this chapter you will have an understanding of the needs of the patient in regard to nutrition and hydration care.

GLOSSARY

Biopsychosocial model of care

An holistic approach to health care incorporating biology, psychology and sociology, referred to as the physical, psychological, sociocultural, environmental and politicoeconomic elements of care.

Adequate nutrition and hydration are essential for health and well-being. This is not rocket science! Florence Nightingale, in her *Notes on Nursing*, some 160 years ago, wrote that '...thousands of patients are annually starved in the midst of plenty' (Nightingale 1860).

In today's more technological world of medical advances, research and education we are still seeing headlines such as 'Hundreds of patients dying of thirst in Britain's hospitals' (Daily Telegraph 2012).

So what is going wrong with the basic nursing care in our hospitals and the community? Not every death related to poor nutrition or hydration can be blamed on poor patient care, as some illnesses such as certain forms of cancer may make it impossible for patients to eat and drink. But according to the Office for National Statistics (2010) the majority of such cases are indeed down to poor care issues.

Let's start with the basics and look at the factors influencing eating and drinking according to the biopsychosocial model of care.

Activity 11.1

Look at Table 11.1 and write down as many factors as you can think of that affect eating and drinking using the biopsychosocial model of care.

Table 11.1 Factors influencing eating and drinking

Biopsychosocial element	Factors (try to put at least three in each section)
Physical	
Psychological	
Sociocultural	
Environmental	
Politicoeconomic	

Adapted from Roper (2000).

NUTRITION

Maintaining an adequate nutritional intake is essential for health and well-being. During times of illness and disease the body's requirement for nutrients is increased to help it recover from infection, trauma, surgery and disease, and to promote wound healing for repair and recovery. Good nutrition is also essential for physiological and psychological well-being.

It is also important to maintain a balanced diet. A balanced, varied diet can help prevent or manage many medical conditions, such as coronary heart disease, obesity, hypertension, stroke and diabetes (National Patient Safety Agency 2009a). It consists of eating a variety of foods in the correct proportions, from each of the five major food categories:

- fruit and vegetables: 33%,
- complex carbohydrates (bread, other cereals and potatoes): 33%,

- proteins (meat, fish and alternatives): 12%,
- milk and diary products: 15%,
- fats and sugars: 7%.

The Royal College of Nursing (2009) has stated that water is also considered to be an essential nutrient, along with carbohydrates, fats, proteins, vitamins and minerals.

Patients being admitted to hospitals and care homes should be assessed to determine their nutritional status – from malnourished to obese – so that if necessary they can be referred to a nutritional expert (e.g. dietician) to plan their care needs during their stay.

Many hospitals and care homes use the Malnutrition Universal Screening Tool (MUST; British Association of Parenteral and Enteral Nutrition 2006), or an adaptation of MUST, on patients and residents as part of the nutritional screening conducted within the first 24 hours of admission. Surveys in the UK inform us that 25% of patients screened during hospital admission were found to be at risk of malnutrition. Forty-one per cent of those screened during admission to care homes were found to be malnourished and 19% of new admissions to mental health units were also malnourished (British Association of Parenteral and Enteral Nutrition 2011). Malnourishment equates to delayed recovery, increased length of hospital stay and increased risk of mortality; in short, poor nutritional state can threaten the safety of those in our care in hospital and other care settings.

The National Patient Safety Agency (NPSA) has compiled a list of key themes that have a bearing on nutritional care, based on observed incidences (see Table 11.2).

As part of the nutritional assessment it may be decided that a patient's nutritional intake should be recorded. A fluid chart may also be commenced to establish fluid balance. It is the nurse's role to ensure that these documents are completed correctly. A multidisciplinary team approach may be initiated, requiring the services of the enteral nutrition team, social workers, key worker/care staff, medical staff, nursing staff, dieticians, speech and

Table 11.2 Key themes relating to nutritional care in hospital according to the NPSA

Theme	Details
Choking	Patients or service users witnessing choking
Dehydration	Intravenous fluids prescribed but not administered
Nil by mouth	Hospital patients being kept nil by mouth for prolonged periods of time
Inappropriate diet	Patients or service users receiving incorrect diets (e.g. food they are allergic to, not providing modified diet for those with swallowing difficulties, etc.)
Catering services	Catering services providing meals at inappropriate temperatures and/or being unable to provide correct diets
Incorrect artificial nutrition	Incorrect doses of artificial nutrition being given
Missed meals	Hospital patients missing meals, e.g. for non-urgent investigations, etc.
Transfer of care	Hospital patients being transferred to care homes, etc. without information relating to their nutritional requirements
Pressure ulcers	Nutrient intake being a contributory factor in the development of pressure ulcers

Data from National Patient Safety Agency (2009b).

language therapists, pharmacists, biochemists, catering staff, domiciliary staff, etc.

Initiatives have been implemented to enable patients to enjoy their meals in an environment conducive to eating – known as protected mealtimes – without the disturbance and noise of visitors, ward rounds, diagnostic tests, etc. This better enables staff to continue to assess and monitor and assist patients in their needs, e.g. physically assisting people to eat their meals and monitoring for swallowing difficulties. If a nurse or carer is unable to take part in the nutritional care of a patient, and this task has been delegated to a relative or assistant, it is the nurse's responsibility to ensure that intake is sufficient for health and to record the intake. It is a very sad state of affairs that nurses are unable to 'nurse' those they are caring for and indeed have to delegate some caring tasks, such as feeding.

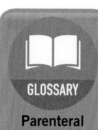

GLOSSARY

Parenteral nutrition (PN)

The giving of nutrients intravenously rather than via the mouth or stomach. This may be in addition to eating food by mouth.

Total parenteral nutrition (TPN)

The practice of solely giving nutrients intravenously rather than via the mouth or stomach, with no additional source of nutrition.

Individuals with swallowing difficulties, after assessment, may require their nutrition in liquid form directly into the stomach, known as enteral nutrition. The food is administered through a hollow tube that goes via either the nose (nasogastric tube) or the mouth (orogastric tube) and down into the stomach. Other tubes can be used to deliver the liquid feed via the jejunal route.

PARENTERAL NUTRITION

Parenteral nutrition (PN) may be initiated for those unable to eat normally and so who cannot receive an adequate nutritional intake to maintain their health, and for those not able to absorb enough nourishment due to illness or disease. PN is delivered through a tube called a central venous catheter (CVC) into a large vein, such as the subclavian vein just above the clavicle. Some devices are known as peripherally inserted central catheter lines (PICC lines) or Hickman lines.

PN solution contains glucose (for energy), proteins (for growth and repair), fat (for energy and cell repair) and vitamins and minerals (to maintain bodily health). Close monitoring for signs of line infection and tolerance of the feed is maintained by:

- observation (temperature, blood pressure, pulse and respiration rate),
- blood tests (to check electrolyte levels and kidney and liver function),
- urine samples,
- body weight,
- blood glucose sample.

KEY ASPECTS OF PROVIDING A CONDUCIVE EATING ENVIRONMENT

Providing patients and service users with optimal nutritional care is an integral part of their treatment and providing for their health needs. As a nurse assisting patients to eat was one of the most enjoyable parts of my working day, engaging those I cared for in conversation and getting to know their hopes and fears, likes and dislikes, etc. On a Sunday we often played music at mealtimes, although this can prove problematic, with some wanting classical music and others wanting more modern sounds! Some of the key aspects of providing a protective mealtime, according to the NPSA (National Patient Safety Agency 2009b), are as follows:

- positioning the patient/service user in an optimal position ready for their meal,
- providing appropriate equipment, e.g. adapted cutlery,
- making sure that individuals have plates and drinks placed close enough to reach,
- ensuring that dentures are in place (and clean)and that dental care is not problematic,
- getting the patient to be involved in choosing their meal and portion size,
- washing the patients hands prior to the meal,
- clearing clutter from table tops,
- making the meal time a social event with other patients, if able,
- enabling those who prefer sitting alone to be alone,
- providing assistance with opening packages,
- assisting those who require it to eat their meal,
- monitoring for swallowing difficulties,
- ensuring adequate nutrition is being ingested,
- ensuring the patient has a drink with their meal (they may require this for extra lubrication if their saliva is diminished),
- recording nutritional intake, if required.

HYDRATION

Water is essential for life and essential for all the body's processes. As well as considering a patient's nutritional requirements it is also vital to ensure that those we care for receive adequate amounts to drink. NHS Choices (2011) recommend that patients should drink up to 2.5 litres of water a day. Water makes up approximately 60–65% of an adult's total body weight. In newborn infants water comprises about 75% of body weight, but this proportion decreases progressively with age after about 3–5 years of age. In early old age the level gradually decreases again.

CHILDREN

Adequate fluid intake is particularly important for children due to their immature thirst mechanisms, high activity levels and high fluid loss due to a large ratio of surface area to body mass. The fluid requirements of children vary with size, age and gender, with girls having a slightly higher percentage of body fat and storing less water than boys.

Table 11.3 shows the suggested daily fluid intake by age and gender according to the National Institute for Health and Clinical Excellence (2010).

Table 11.3 Daily fluid intake recommendations for children

Age	Total per day (mL)	
	Male	Female
4–8 years	1000–1400 mL	1000–1400 mL
9–13 years	1400–2300 mL	1200–2100 mL
14–18 years	2100–3200 mL	1400–2500 mL

The kidneys remove waste from the body as urine and play an important part in regulating fluid balance, functioning better in the presence of an adequate fluid supply. A good fluid intake also helps to establish day and night bladder control due to the fact that as bladder capacity is increased the child learns to understand the feeling of a full bladder and the fact that they need to go for a 'wee'.

GOOD HYDRATION IN THE OLDER PATIENT

Many older people do not drink adequate amounts of water. This may be due to cognitive impairment, changes in functional ability, medications or stress arising from other factors (Water UK 2005). Coupled with this is the fact that as we get older the kidneys' vital role in regulating the amount of fluid in the body diminishes. Dehydration has been identified as one of the risk factors for falls in older people, due to it leading to a deterioration in mental state and an increased risk of dizziness and fainting. The benefits of good hydration in older people are summarised below.

Pressure ulcers   Poorly hydrated individuals are twice as likely to experience pressure ulcers. Increased hydration can increase levels of oxygenation and enhance ulcer healing.

Constipation   Poor hydration is one of the most frequent causes of constipation. Good hydration can increase stool frequency and enhance the effects of dietary fibre.

Urinary tract infections and continence   Water helps to maintain a healthy urinary tract and kidneys.

Kidney and gallstones   Good hydration can reduce the risk of kidney-stone formation and gallstone formation.

Heart disease   Good hydration reduces the risk of coronary heart disease and also protects against blood-clot formation by decreasing blood viscosity.

Low blood pressure   Drinking a glass of water before standing can prevent fainting due to low blood pressure, which many older people experience.

Diabetes   Dehydration can worsen diabetic control, with good hydration helping to maintain healthy blood sugar levels.

Cognitive impairment   Dehydration can reduce alertness and the ability to concentrate.

INTRACELLULAR AND EXTRACELLULAR FLUIDS AND ELECTROLYTES

Bodily water is distributed between two major reservoirs or spaces: the **intracellular** and **extracellular** compartments, separated by a cellular semipermeable membrane. The extracellular fluid compartment is subdivided into **interstitial fluid** and **plasma**. In the body fluid are electrically charged atoms or ions called electrolytes, which have an important impact on electrochemical and osmotic activity within each fluid compartment. Water moves from an area of lesser osmotic pressure to one of greater osmotic pressure until an equilibrium has been reached. This is explained more fully in chapter 10 of *Medicine Management Skills for Nurses* in the Student Survival Skills Series (Boyd 2013). Concentrations of electrolytes in serum can be seen in Table 11.4.

Table 11.4 Concentrations of electrolytes in serum

Electrolyte	Normal range
Sodium	135–145 mmol/L
Chloride	95–105 mmol/L
Potassium	3.3–5.0 mmol/L
Hydrogen carbonate (bicarbonate)	22–30 mmol/L
Calcium	2.12–2.65 mmol/L

Positive Fluid Balance

If diminished excretion occurs with continued intake, resulting in excessive volume in the fluid compartments, a positive fluid balance occurs. Electrolyte concentrations are changed, with a harmful fluid excess developing and harmful wastes being retained.

Negative Fluid Balance

Fluid loss (due to micturition, diarrhoea, vomiting, sweating, etc.) exceeding fluid input is known as a negative fluid balance. Abnormal fluid shifts occur between the fluid departments, affecting bodily functions and electrolyte readings. Patients with a fluid volume deficit may present with the following clinical characteristics:

- dry skin/mucous membranes,
- increased serum sodium,
- increased pulse rate,
- decreased blood pressure,
- decreased or excessive urine output,
- concentrated urine or urine frequency,
- decreased fluid intake,
- decreased skin turgor,

- thirst/nausea/anorexia,
- weakness/lethargy,
- decreased level of concentration,
- decreased level of consciousness.

FLUID REPLACEMENT

Fluid and electrolyte replacement may consist of the parenteral fluids found in Table 11.5.

Table 11.5 Parenteral fluids for fluid and electrolyte replacement

Fluid	Details, benefits
Mannitol	Inert form of sugar mannose; used to raise intravascular volume and to increase urinary output
Sodium chloride 0.9%	Used to replace body fluid; also to raise plasma volume when red blood cell mass is adequate. Increases plasma volume without altering normal sodium concentration or serum osmolarity
Hartmann's solution	0.9% Sodium chloride with added electrolytes; used to replace body fluid and to buffer acidosis
Ringer's solution	0.9% Sodium chloride in water with added potassium and calcium; used to replace body fluid. Also used to provide additional potassium and calcium
Dextrose 5%	5% Dextrose in water; used to raise total fluid volume. Distributed evenly in every body compartment
Sodium chloride 0.45%	0.45% Sodium chloride in water; used to raise total fluid volume

Adequate nutrition and hydration are vital for health and well-being, and they encroach on every aspect of the biopsychosocial model of care. As thirst is a late presentation of dehydration, cool, fresh water should be offered at regular intervals in the care setting, and placed within easy reach.

However, it should be remembered that some patients will have fluid restrictions as a result of their medical condition, with limits to the amount of fluid that they can drink. For example, in the initial stages of treatment for pancreatitis only hourly sips of water are to be tolerated.

TEST YOUR KNOWLEDGE

1 Mrs Brady has been admitted to your clinical area and had blood taken for biochemistry testing. The medic informs us that Mrs Brady is severely dehydrated. What clinical characteristics would she be showing?
2 How much fluid should a boy aged 14–18 years drink in 24 hours?
3 What is the normal range of the electrolyte sodium in an adult?
4 What are the components of a balanced diet?

KEY POINTS

- The biopsychosocial model of care.
- Nutritional components of a balanced diet.
- NPSA themes relating to nutritional care in the hospital environment.
- Parenteral nutrition.
- Providing a conducive eating environment.
- Hydration: issues in children and the older patient.
- Intracellular and extracellular fluids and electrolytes.
- Fluid replacement.

Bibliography

Age Concern (2006) *Hungry To be Heard*. Age Concern, London.

Alzheimer's Society (2012) *Eating*. http://www.alzheimers.org.uk/site/scripts/documents.php?categoryID=200367.

Archibald, C. (2006a) Meeting the nutritional needs of patients with dementia in hospital. *Nursing Standard* 20(45), 41–45.

Archibald, C. (2006b) Promoting hydration in patients with dementia in healthcare settings. *Nursing Standard*, 20(44), 49–52.

Bloomfield, J. and Pegram, A. (2012) Improving nutrition and hydration in hospital: the nurse's responsibility. *Nursing Standard* 26(34), 52–56.

Boyd, C. (2013) *Medicine Management Skills for Nurses*. Wiley Blackwell, Oxford.

British Association of Parenteral and Enteral Nutrition (2006) *Malnutrition Universal Screening Tool*. www.bapen.org.uk

British Association of Parenteral and Enteral Nutrition (2011) *The Nutritional Screening Survey.* www.bapen.org.uk

Daily Telegraph (2012) Hundreds of patients dying of thirst in Britain's hospitals. www.telegraph.co.uk/health/healthnews/9549883/Hundreds-of-patients-dying-of-thirst-in-Britains-hospitals.html.

Jacques, E. (2012) Promoting healthy drinking habits in children. *Nursing Times* 108(41), 20–21.

National Institute for Health and Clinical Excellence (2010) *Nocturnal Enuresis: the Management of Bedwetting in Children and Young People.* Clinical Guideline CG111. www.nice.org.uk/CG111.

National Patient Safety Agency (2009a) *The Care Provider has a Policy for Food Service and Nutritional care, Which is Centred on the Needs of Users, and is Performance Managed in Line with Home Country Governance and/or Regulatory Framework.* Fact Sheet 10. www.nrls.npsa.nhs.uk/EasySiteWeb/getresource.axd?AssetID=60241&.

National Patient Safety Agency (2009b) Food Service and Nutritional Care is Delivered Safety. Fact Sheet 1. www.nrls.npsa.nhs.uk/EasySiteWeb/getresource.axd?AssetID=60229&.

NHS Choices (2011) *Water and Drinks.* www.nhs.uk/Livewell/Goodfood/Pages/water-drinks.aspx.

Nightingale, F. (1860) *Notes on Nursing – What it is and What it is Not.* Reprinted by Dover Publications, New York.

Office of National Statistics (2010) *United Kingdom Health Statistics*, 48th edn. www.ons.gov.uk

Roper, N., Logan, W. and Tierney, A.J. (2000) *The Elements of Nursing: a Model for Nursing Based on a Model of Living*, 4th edn. Elsevier Health Sciences, Edinburgh.

Royal College of Nursing (2009) *Hospital Hydration Best Practice Toolkit.* http://tinyurl.com/6t3c5xr.

Water UK (2005) *Wise up on Water! Hydration and Healthy Ageing.* www.water.org.uk/home/news/press-releases/wise-up-on-water/wise-up—older.pdf?s1=older+people

Chapter 12
. . . .
WOUND CARE

Care Skills for Nurses, First Edition. Claire Boyd
© 2014 John Wiley & Sons, Ltd. Published 2014 by John Wiley & Sons, Ltd.

LEARNING OUTCOMES

By the end of this chapter you will be have a better understanding of wound management.

Wound care management is a vast subject in its own right and this chapter only seeks to skim the basics of the topic. Before we start, let's get our head around some of the terminology associated with wound care.

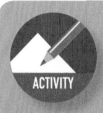

Activity 12.1

ACTIVITY

What do these terms mean?

1 Necrotic
2 Sloughy
3 Granulating
4 Epithelialising
5 Macerated skin
6 Debridement

WOUND CARE PREVENTION

In order to prevent wound care problems, the following issues need to be considered in wound management:

- skin inspection,
- moisture control,
- correct manual handling techniques,
- assessing nutritional and fluid intake,
- avoiding pressure on heels and bony prominences,
- correct use of positioning devices,
- good documentation, monitoring and reporting.

THE SKIN

The skin is the largest organ of the body; it covers the body's surface in a continuous layer of tissue.

Question 12.1   What basic 'skin test' can we perform to establish whether someone is dehydrated?

The skin acts as a defensive organ against outside factors and also as a protector of the internal organs. It is a barrier against infection. Intact it prevents bacteria and micro-organisms from entering the body (other aspects of the skin's structure and function are described in Chapters 3 and 5).

The skin has two main parts: the epidermis and the dermis. Under these layers is the subcutaneous layer.

The Epidermis

Stratum corneum   The uppermost layer or surface layer (stratified epithelium), which is made of hard, flattened dead cells which are constantly being shed. In these cells the cytoplasm is replaced by keratin, which waterproofs the skin. As these cells are rubbed off with daily living, by clothes and by rubbing the skin's surface, they are replaced from below. It is said that we shed between 18 and 23 kg of skin cells in our lifetime! There are areas of various thicknesses: for example, the thickest areas are found on the soles of the feet and the palms of the hands. The thinnest areas are found on the eyelids and the nipples. The fingerprints, unique to each individual, including twins, are made up of papillary ridges.

Stratum lucidum   This is a clear layer of denucleated cells (i.e. without a nucleus). They are not completely hard and the cell membranes can be seen under a microscope from skin of the palms and soles.

Stratum granulosum   This is known as the granular layer, in which the cells are dying but still have a nucleus. This is visible following a trauma to the skin and is the tissue that is healing.

Stratum spinosum   The prickle cell layer; the cells are living and the membranes are intact with interlocking fibrils. These cells are capable of mitosis (division and replication), especially on the palms and soles where hard skin is produced for protection.

Stratum germinativum   The basal layer. By its name you can see it is the bottom layer of the epidermis and this is where cell division takes place. It takes about 28–30 days for the cells to move up through the five layers before they are shed (except in the condition psoriasis, where the cells move up within 3–4 days, giving the scaly effect). This layer contains the pigment melanin, produced by melanocyte cells, which protects against ultraviolet radiation and gives the skin its colour. This is dependent on the climate and the amount of protection the skin needs, so dark skin will be protected against the sun's rays better than pale skin, which will burn easily.

Even though this layer is very fine, it does not contain nerves or blood vessels, which is why we do not bleed from a paper cut. It does, however, contain sweat ducts and hair follicles to allow excretion from the layer below.

The Dermis

This is the layer below the epidermis and is made up of specialised cells of connective tissue; mainly areolar tissue, which is tough and elastic. It has the ability to stretch as we grow outwards and this is due to the white collagen fibres and elastin, which is yellow elastic tissue. These keep the skin supple, but the elasticity and the suppleness tend to diminish as we get older.

The dermis contains capillaries, which are the blood vessels providing the skin with oxygen and nutrients. The living cells of the skin produce waste products such as carbon dioxide and metabolic waste. These products pass from the cells and enter the bloodstream to be taken away and removed from the body.

The Subcutaneous Layer

The subcutaneous layer is situated below the dermis. It consists of adipose tissue (fat) and areolar tissue. The adipose tissue helps to protect the body against injury and acts as an insulating layer against heat loss, helping to keep the body warm. The areolar tissue contains elastic fibres, making this layer elastic and flexible. Muscle is situated below the subcutaneous layer.

WOUNDS: CAUSES AND TYPES

Wounds come in a variety of shapes and sizes and can be either chronic or acute. Just as every patient must be treated as an individual, wounds also need to be treated for their own characteristics and uniqueness.

Wounds occur when the skin is broken and damage may have been caused in a variety of ways, such as:

- **inflammation:** the skin's response to injury,
- **superficial wounds and abrasions:** leaving the deeper skin layers intact; usually caused by abrasion or tears,
- **deep abrasion:** caused by cuts or lacerations; these go through all the layers of the skin and into underlying tissues such as muscle or bone,
- **puncture wounds:** usually caused by sharp pointed objects puncturing the skin,
- **pressure sores:** usually caused by sitting or lying too long in the same position; tissue death occurs due to lack of blood supply in the area of skin under pressure,
- **burns.**

Wounds can also be categorised as being caused by:

- pressure ulcers,
- arterial insufficiency,
- diabetic ulcers,
- venous insufficiency,
- surgical wounds,
- tumours,
- trauma,

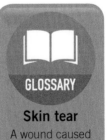

GLOSSARY

Skin tear
A wound caused by shear, friction and/or blunt force that results in separation of the skin layers. This type of injury usually occurs in immature skin (neonates) and older people.

- skin tears,
- burns.

CLASSIFICATION OF WOUNDS

There are many wound care classification systems available, such as the European Pressure Ulcer Advisory Panel classification system (as seen in Chapter 5) specifically for pressure ulcer grading. These grading systems are beneficial as they allow the carer to continually assess a wound and the effects of the treatment programme.

Whichever system is used, it should record both the type of tissue present and the stage of the wound healing process, which are:

- dry and necrotic,
- sloughy/necrotic,
- clean and granulating,
- epithelialising,
- infected.

WOUND COLOUR CODING

Colour coding is also a useful tool to aid interpretation of the wound healing process.

ACTIVITY

Activity 12.2

What colour of tissue would you expect to see with each of these wound terms?

Necrotic
Sloughy
Granulating
Epithelialising
Infected

WOUND HEALING

The stages of wound healing are:

- acute/traumatic inflammation and destructive phase (takes approximately 0–6 days),
- proliferative phase (takes approximately 3–,4 days),
- maturation (can take months).

The inflammatory and proliferative stages take place concurrently.

Wound Healing by First Intention

This is the rapid, primary healing process. An example of this is in clean surgical incisions where the wound edges are in apposition. Staples or stitches may be used for this type of wound closure. Wound healing by first intention occurs due to the following factors:

- a blood clot fills the wound and the inflammatory response is initiated,
- neutrophils and macrophages clear away the clot and cellular debris,
- macrophages stimulate the development of fibroblasts and secrete collagen,
- granulation tissue is formed from the collagen and newly formed capillaries; the new tissue and capillaries fill the gap,
- epidermal cells regenerate from the wound edges and grow across the granulation tissue; this process is called epithelialisation,
- when epithelialisation is complete the scab is dislodged; the wound continues to repair and strengthen and usually reaches full strength after about 3 months.

Wound Healing by Second Intention

Wound healing by second intention is where there is tissue loss and healing occurs slowly as the cavity heals from the bottom up. An example of this is in pressure sores or gaping wounds:

- infection must be overcome by the inflammatory response,
- necrotic tissue is removed,
- foreign bodies must be removed,
- granulating tissue starts at the floor of the cavity and takes much longer to commence initially,
- epithelialisation takes longer to occur,
- the fibrous scar will be larger due to the wound edges not being in apposition.

Wound Cleaning

Wounds should be cleaned to remove any debris and a moist environment should be maintained. Necrotic tissue should be softened and the wound debrided. A strict aseptic approach should be maintained to decrease the risk of bacterial contamination. An assessment of wound appearance, depth and size should be conducted and documented and the correct dressing should then be obtained.

Factors Known to Influence Wound Healing

The following factors are known to delay the wound healing process:

- infection,
- poor blood supply, e.g. cardiovascular disease,
- foreign bodies in the wound and the presence of necrosis,
- diabetes mellitus,
- poor nutritional status,
- widespread malignancy and immune problems,
- repeated wound trauma,
- inappropriate dressings,
- stress (with high corticosteroid levels),
- cigarette smoking.

Factors Known to Promote the Wound Healing Process

Adequate nutrition will assist the wound healing process. Here are some of the main nutrients involved:

- carbohydrates: used in the inflammatory response,
- protein: used in the synthesis of new tissue,
- fats: used in the formation of inflammatory mediators and clotting components,
- zinc: used in cell growth,
- manganese, copper, selenium: important in enzymic and oxidation processes during the wound healing process,
- iron: used in the transport of oxygen,
- vitamin A: important in the inflammatory response and for wound strength,
- vitamin B_1: collagen for cellular activity,
- vitamin C: increases wound strength,
- vitamin E: haemostasis (slows blood flow).

OVERVIEW OF WOUND CARE PRODUCTS

After assessment, the best wound care product will need to be obtained for the patient's wound. It should be remembered that when dressing wounds the patient may experience pain and/or discomfort. It is always best to consider pain relief prior to starting the procedure. Some patients may prefer a non-medicinal approach to their pain management, such as distraction.

Some of the products on the market, and their indications for use, are shown in Table 12.1. Products are continuously being developed, however, and new research articles published – such as about the use of mannuka honey in wound healing – so this is not an exhaustive list from the Wound Care Formulary (included in the *British National Formulary*).

Table 12.1 Dressing products and their indications for use

Product	Indications for use
Alginates	Used in the management of heavily exuding wounds; has haemostatic properties (stops bleeding)
Cadexomer iodine	Used in the treatment of chronic exuding wounds, particularly when an infection is present or suspected
Hydrocolloids	Used on many wound types and granulating wounds; as the debris is removed, sloughy wounds will appear larger initially
Hydrofibre	Used in the treatment of exuding wounds, including donor sites and first- and second-degree burns; also used in surgical or traumatic wounds
Hydrogels	Used to treat dry sloughy or necrotic wounds; also used for cavity wounds and infected wounds
Metronidazole	Used as a deodoriser in the management of malodorous fungating tumours
Non-adherent or low-adherence dressing	Used in the management of clean, lightly exuding, superficial wounds; reduces trauma during dressing change
Non-adherent silicone foam dressing	Used in many types of exuding wounds, such as pressure ulcers and traumatic wounds resulting in skin loss; can also be used under compression bandaging
Odour-absorbing dressings	These dressings can be placed directly on to the wound or placed over an existing primary dressing
Polyurethane foam dressing	Used on a variety of exuding wounds; keeps the exudate locked away, thus preventing maceration
Povidone-iodine sheet	Indicated for the prophylaxis and treatment of wound infection
Protease-modulating matrix	Used in the management of all types of chronic wounds that are free of necrotic tissue and visible signs of infection
Rapid capillary dressing	Used in the treatment of a wide range of wounds from minor to chronic, wet or dry

Product	Indications for use
Semi-permeable adhesive film dressing	Used in the management of shallow wounds, minor burns, donor sites, post-operative wounds, abrasions and minor lacerations
Soft silicone dressing	Used in the treatment of skin tears, abrasions and in blistering skin conditions; also used for skin damage following radiotherapy or steroid therapy
Silver dressings	Used to decontaminate wounds and inhibit the growth of certain bacteria

Data from British National Formulary (2010).

SPECIALIST PRODUCTS

Specialist products used in wound care include those listed in Table 12.2.

Table 12.2 Specialist wound care products

Product	Key characteristics
Larvae (also known as 'maggot therapy')	Used to debride sloughy, necrotic or infected wounds
Vacuum-assisted closure (also known as negative pressure treatment)	The vacuum-assisted closure device is used to assist drainage of blood or serous fluid from a wound or operation site; it is used to treat diabetic foot ulcers, acute and traumatic wounds, pressure ulcers and chronic open wounds
VEC high-compression bandage	Used to apply controlled levels of pressure in the treatment of venous ulcers

TEST YOUR KNOWLEDGE

1 What does debride mean?
2 List the ways in which wounds can be categorised.
3 What factors are known to delay the wound healing process?
4 What are hydrogel dressings used for?
5 What are the indications for the use of larvae therapy?
6 What does the term haemostatic properties mean?

KEY POINTS

- The skin.
- Causes and types of wound.
- Wound healing.
- Factors known to delay the wound healing process.
- Overview of wound care products.

Bibliography

Alexander, S. (2009) Malignant fungating wounds: managing pain, bleeding and psychosocial issues. *Journal of Wound Care* 18(10), 418–425.

Beldon, P. (2006) Topical negative pressure dressings and vacuum-assisted closure. *Wound Essentials* 1, 110–114.

Blanchi, J. (2012) Preventing, assessing and managing skin tears. *Nursing Times* 108(13), 12–14.

Boulton, A.J.M. and Vileikyte, L. (2000) The diabetic foot. The scope of the problem. *Journal of Family Practice* 49(11), S3–S8.

Bowler, P.G., Duerden, B.I. and Armstrong, D.G. (2001) Wound microbiology and associated approaches to wound management. *Clinical Microbiology Reviews* 14(2), 244–269.

British National Formulary (2010) *British National Formulary No 59*. British Medical Association and Royal Pharmaceutical Society of Great Britain, London.

Dougherty, L. and Lister, S. (eds) (2011) *The Royal Marsden Hospital Manual of Clinical Nursing Procedures*, 8th edn. Wiley-Blackwell, Oxford.

Flanagan, M. (2000) The physiology of wound healing. *Journal of Wound Care* 9(6), 299–300.

Garrett, B. (1997) The proliferation and movement of cells during re-epithelialisation. *Journal of Wound Care* 6(4), 174–177.

Grocott, P. (2007) Care of patients with fungating malignant wounds. *Nursing Standard* 21(24), 57–58, 60, 62 passim.

Hampton, S. (2008) Malodorous fungating wounds: how dressings alleviate symptoms. *British Journal of Community Nursing* 13(6), S31–S32, S34, S36 passim.

Maylor, M.E. (2001) Accurate selection of compression and antiembolic hosiery. *British Journal of Nursing* 10(18), 1172–1184.

Northern Health and Social Services Board (2005) *NHSSB Wound Management Manual*. www.nhssb.n-i.nhs.uk/publications/primary_care/Wound_Manual.pdf.

Thomas, S. (2009) *Formulary of Wound Management Products*, 10th edn. Euromed Communications, Liphook.

White, R. (2001) Managing exudate. *Nursing Times* 97(14), 59–60.

Wolcott, R.D., Kennedy, J.P. and Dowd, S.E. (2009) Regular debridement is the main tool for maintaining a healthy wound bed in most chronic wounds. *Journal of Wound Care* 18(92), 54–56.

Answers to Activities, Questions and Test Your Knowledge

CHAPTER 1

Activity 1.1

- Sarah is in pain: why has no one considered pain relief for her?
- Why has her nicotine dependence not been addressed, i.e. with nicotine patches or referral to a smoking-cessation clinic?
- Why did someone else not see to Sarah's urgent toileting requirements? How very undignified for Sarah to have passed urine in the bed and all over herself.
- How was the fact that you were busy explained to Sarah and how long did she have to wait?
- Never tut at a patient: this is very unprofessional.
- In summary, very little care and compassion has been shown to Sarah.

Activity 1.2

1 Communication
2 Toileting
3 Pain relief
4 Nutrition and hydration

Chapter 1 Test Your Knowledge

1 Care, compassion, competence, communication, courage, commitment

CHAPTER 2

Chapter 2 Questions

2.1 These micro-organisms are usually spread from person to person in the following ways: (1) by direct contact, such as the hands, (2) by equipment, instruments and cloths, (3) via blood and body fluids, (4) via the faecal/oral route, (5) by particles and droplets in the atmosphere (airborne), (6) via animal vectors.

2.2 (1) Prior to performing any invasive procedures, such as catheter care or administering eye drops, (2) after bed making, (3) before food preparation, (4) when hands are visibly soiled or just when they feel dirty, (5) after contact with

Care Skills for Nurses, First Edition. Claire Boyd
© 2014 John Wiley & Sons, Ltd. Published 2014 by John Wiley & Sons, Ltd.

a patient, (6) before putting on gloves, (7) after taking off gloves, (8) after going to the toilet, (9) after providing hygiene care or toilet care to a service user, (10) when they have not been washed for some time.

2.3 A selection of some of the times gloves should be worn: (1) when dealing with body fluids, (2) if you have any skin breaks or openings (which should be covered), (3) when dealing with chemicals, (4) when decontaminating equipment, (5) if there is any infectious risk from the patient, (6) as a precaution, after conducting a risk assessment, (7) to prevent cross-infection, (8) during any aseptic procedure (sterile gloves), (9) when preparing food (vinyl gloves), (10) when preparing medications, such as reconstituting freeze-dried antibiotics, etc.

Chapter 2 Test Your Knowledge

1 Before patient contact, before an aseptic task, after body-fluid exposure, after patient contact, after contact with patient surroundings.

2 Tips of fingers, between fingers and around thumb.

3 Wearing rings and watches around the wrist increases the number of bacteria on the hands.

4 The six-point hand-wash technique.

5 The same: the six-point hand-wash technique.

6 This is a new strain of MRSA, first discovered in the USA, which has the appearance of a spider bite.

CHAPTER 3

Chapter 3 Questions

3.1 The skin acts as a defensive organ against outside factors and also as a protector of the internal organs. It is a barrier against infection. Intact it prevents bacteria and micro-organisms from entering the body. It also produces vitamin D, acts in thermoregulation, excretes toxic chemicals, allows us to experience the world by touch and protects us from harmful stimuli.

3.2 (1) Knee-high: these stockings should sit below the knee; (2) thigh-high: the stocking border should rest below the buttocks; (3) waist-high (or pantyhose): these stockings should rest around the waist with the seams turning vertically up the front of the garment.

Chapter 3 Test Your Knowledge

1 Choose from: heat regulation, absorption, excretion, secretion, vitamin D formation, sensation and protection.

2 Knee-high, thigh-high and waist-high (or pantyhose).

3 A thorough inspection of the skin, observing for pressure ulcers, marks, breaks in the skin, bruising etc.; in addition, observation of the patient's pain levels and psychological well-being.

4   c, A chiropodist.

CHAPTER 4

Activity 4.1

a   Deep yellow/orange urine: this could be due to dehydration or jaundice. Bilirubin – the breakdown product of haemoglobin, excreted in bile and in small amounts in urine – may be detected in a urinalysis test. It may also be caused by drugs such as rifampicin.

b   Blue urine: this may be caused by a chemical called Methylene Blue, which is added to fresh frozen plasma (a blood-product transfusion) and administered to neonates and small children. This chemical is added to inactivate any viruses present in this blood product to protect their underdeveloped immune systems. It may also cause temporarily blue skin, the reason why parents may call their baby a 'smurf baby'!

c   Red urine: this may be blood caused by trauma or kidney cancer. It may also be caused by eating large amounts of beetroot, but only temporarily.

d   Blue/green urine: this may be caused by a pseudomonal urine infection. A urinalysis test would show protein in the urine.

Chapter 4 Question

4.1   Urine is mainly made up of water (95%), with the following elements: 0.05% ammonia, 0.18% sulphate, 0.12% phosphate, 0.6% chloride, 0.01% magnesium, 0.015% calcium, 0.6% potassium, 0.1% sodium, 0.1% creatinine, 0.03% uric acid and 2% urea. Protein should not be present in urine.

Chapter 4 Test Your Knowledge

1   The involuntary passing of urine
2   Nocturnal enuresis
3   Stress incontinence, urgency/ urge incontinence, overflow incontinence, reflex incontinence, environmental/locomotor incontinence, functional incontinence
4   Meconium
5   Usual stool consistency, usual stool frequency, pain associated with bowel motion, presence of blood and/or mucus, evacuation problems, past medical history, toilet-access issues, diet and fluid intake, medication, including over-the-counter medications
6   75% water and 25% solid matter

CHAPTER 5

Chapter 5 Questions

5.1
    1   Long periods lying in a bed or sitting in a chair

2 Reduced mobility or immobility, including people in plaster casts, with spinal cord injuries, etc.
3 Old age or infirmity with inactivity
4 Incontinence, faecal and urinary = excess moisture
5 Significant obesity or thinness
6 Poor nutrition
7 Dehydration
8 Diabetes
9 Vascular disease, including stroke and poor circulation
10 Lowered mental awareness
11 Lowered pain awareness
12 Fractures
13 Medication, including sedatives and steroids
14 Carcinoma
15 Previous pressure ulcer
16 Poor manual handling
17 Delayed treatment
18 Infection
19 Anaemia
20 Immunosuppression

5.2 Malleolus: the protuberance on each side of the ankle.
Greater trochanter: the protuberance that occurs below the neck of the femur.

Chapter 5 Test Your Knowledge

1 Low risk = daily
2 Medium risk = 4 hourly
3 Low risk = daily
4 High risk = 2 hourly
5 Medium risk = 4 hourly
6 High risk = 2 hourly

CHAPTER 6

Chapter 6 Questions

6.1 Balance, urinary problems, medication, blood pressure, memory, vision

6.2 Footwear: sloppy slippers, slippery soles, foot care; trip hazards: zimmer frames stacked untidily, commodes left at bedsides inappropriately; risky behaviour: trying to walk when drip stands/catheters are attached to beds, walking without aids; slippery surfaces: wet floors; bed heights/rails: beds being left inappropriately high, rails being put up without proper assessment

6.3 Appropriate footwear, a bell to call for assistance, clean glasses and operational hearing aids, reporting change in vision to a doctor, giving regular assistance for toileting needs, removing bedside clutter, low bed

Chapter 6 Test Your Knowledge

1 Failure to recognise (Early Warning Scores), failure to respond: new observation charts (escalation measures); failure to communicate: SBAR communication tool, or Situation, Background, Assessment, Recommendation
2 More than 36 000 reported in mental health units
3 Physical injuries, loss of independence, fear of falling, social impact, carer impact, cost to services

4 Checking once an hour: specifically, toileting, pain, confusion, comfort/position, offering a drink, reminding the patient about the call bell/ensuring it is in reach, checking bed height, checking rails are down, asking whether anything else is needed

5 Entrapment, and climbing over and falling to the floor

6 Pain, infection, constipation, hydration, medication, environment

3 Irritable bowel syndrome (bowel), ulcerated colitis (bowel), cancer (bowel or urinary), diverticulitis or Crohn's disease (bowel), trauma (bowel or urinary), neurological damage (urinary or bowel), cancer of the pelvis (urinary or bowel), congenital disorder (urinary or bowel).

4 The drainage bag may not stick to the skin if certain commercial preparations are used.

CHAPTER 7

Chapter 7 Questions

7.1 Ileal conduit: this is where the ureters are diverted from the bladder into a new 'bladder sac', usually part of the bowel: the new ileal conduit. The other end of the ileal conduit opens onto the surface of the skin: the stoma.
Nephrostomy: this is where a long tube is placed straight into the kidney. At the other end of the tube a collection bag is attached for urine drainage.

7.2 Large bowel diversion = colostomy; small bowel diversion = ileostomy; urinary diversion = urostomy, ileal conduit or nephrostomy

Chapter 7 Test Your Knowledge

1 Urostomy, ileal conduit or nephrostomy.

2 The area of skin around the stoma site.

CHAPTER 8

Chapter 8 Questions

8.1 Temperature, pulse, respiratory rate, blood pressure, oxygen saturations, blood glucose

8.2 A DVT is a deep-vein thrombosis, the most common form of VTE.

8.3 This is a pump containing insulin that administers the drug to the patient intravenously to tightly regulate the blood glucose levels. Blood glucose levels are checked, usually hourly to two hourly, by finger-prick capillary glucose monitoring machines and the pump is then titrated accordingly to deliver the correct amount of medication.

Chapter 8 Test Your Knowledge

1 Pre-operative, intra-operative, post-operative

2 General anaesthetic (GA), regional block (such as spinal block,

epidural or nerve block), local anaesthetic
3   Assessment, nursing diagnosis, planning, implementation, evaluation
4   2: intake of water and other clear fluid up to 2 hours before induction of anaesthesia; 4: breast milk up to 4 hours before; 6: formula milk, cow's milk or solids up to 6 hours before
5   It should be stopped 24 hours pre-operatively.
6   Operating department practitioner

CHAPTER 9

Chapter 9 Questions

9.1 Foods, injected venom, drugs, latex
9.2 Cephalosporin antibiotics: a group of semi-synthetic antibiotics derived from the mould *Cephalosporium*. Used to treat a variety of infections.
Sulpha antibiotics: derived from sulphanilamide, which prevents the growth of bacteria.
Allopurinol: a drug used in the treatment of gout by reducing the level of uric acid in the blood and tissues.
9.3 No. Patients with anaphylaxis can deteriorate if made to sit up or stand up. Lie the patient down and raise their feet.

Chapter 9 Test Your Knowledge

1   Food
2   Drugs

3   Swelling to the facial area (mouth and throat) and neck. May cause laryngeal oedema, if severe enough, and airway obstruction.
4   Allergic rash: red wheals develop on the skin. They may itch profusely and last for hours or days.
5   During anaphylaxis, the blood vessels leak, bronchial tissues swell and the blood pressure drops, causing the choking and collapse. Adrenaline acts to constrict blood vessels, relax the smooth muscles in the lungs, stimulates heart contractility and help stop swelling around the face and lips (angio-oedema).
6   Peanuts, tree nuts (walnuts, pecans, pistachios, cob nuts, cashews, almonds), shellfish, fish, milk, pulses (lentils), sesame, soy, wheat, eggs, some fruit and vegetables

CHAPTER 10

Chapter 10 Test Your Knowledge

1   b
2   d
3   a, b
4   c

CHAPTER 11

Activity 11.1

Physical: illness, poor state of mouth and teeth, swallowing difficulties, unable to shop/prepare food, unable to eat food/drink without assistance from individuals/special utensils, depression, unable to respond/recognise appetite/thirst triggers

Psychological: do not have intellectual capabilities to shop/prepare food and drink, do not have intellectual capabilities of nutritional needs, distorted body image, 'comfort' eating/emotional issues, possibly with malnutrition or obesity, alcohol dependence, likes and dislikes, do not have intellectual capabilities to store food, change of diet/routine

Sociocultural: family traditions, religious restrictions, cultural factors, beliefs/values e.g. vegetarianism/veganism

Environmental: means of cooking, means of storage, climate, facilities to procure food, facilities for growing food, distance from home to shopping area

Politicoeconomic: malnutrition, obesity, poor finances, choice of food and drink, quantity and quality of food and drink, safe food (government warnings over contaminated foods etc.)

Chapter 11 Test Your Knowledge

1   Dry skin/mucous membranes, increased serum sodium, increased pulse rate, decreased blood pressure, decreased or excessive urine output, concentrated urine or urine frequency, decreased fluid intake, decreased skin turgor, thirst/nausea/anorexia, weakness/lethargy, decreased level of concentration, decreased level of consciousness

2   2100–3200 mL
3   135–145 mmol/L
4   Fruit and vegetables (33%), complex carbohydrates (bread, other cereals and potatoes; 33%), proteins (meat, fish and alternatives; 12%), milk and diary products (15%), fats and sugars (7%)

CHAPTER 12

Activity 12.1

1   Necrotic: dead tissue
2   Sloughy: dead tissue, a viscous layer that adheres to the wound
3   Granulating: the process by which the wound is filled with highly vascular fragile connective tissue
4   Epithelialising: the process by which the wound is covered with new skin cells
5   Macerated skin: a softening or sogginess of surrounding tissue
6   Debridement: removal of dead, contaminated, infected tissue or any foreign matter from the wound site

Activity 12.2

Necrotic: black
Sloughy: cream/yellow
Granulating: red
Epithelialising: pink
Infected: green

Chapter 12 Question

12.1 The skin may lack its normal elasticity and revert to its usual position only slowly when pinched gently into a fold; this shows a lack of skin turgor. In a hydrated person the skin springs back into position. Care must be taken not to harm the person when trying to make an assessment and diagnosis.

Chapter 12 Test Your Knowledge

1   Removal of dead, contaminated, infected tissue or any foreign matter from the wound site

2   Pressure ulcers, arterial insufficiency, diabetic ulcers, venous insufficiency, surgical wounds, tumours, trauma, skin tears, burns

3   Infection, poor blood supply e.g. cardiovascular disease, foreign bodies in the wound and the presence of necrosis, diabetes mellitus, poor nutritional status, widespread malignancy and immune problems, repeated wound trauma, inappropriate dressings, stress (with high corticosteroid levels), cigarette smoking

4   They are used to treat dry sloughy or necrotic wounds. They are also used for cavity wounds and infected wounds.

5   The need to debride sloughy, necrotic or infected wounds

6   It means that it stops bleeding

Appendix 1

THE COMPONENTS OF MEDICAL WORDS AND TERMS

Care Skills for Nurses, First Edition. Claire Boyd
© 2014 John Wiley & Sons, Ltd. Published 2014 by John Wiley & Sons, Ltd.

Component	Meaning	Example
a-/an-	without, lack of	aphasic (lack of breathing)
ab-	away from	abduction (moving a limb away from the body)
ad-	towards	adduction (moving a limb towards the body)
aer-	air	aerobic (requiring oxygen)
-aesthesia	sensation	paraesthesia (disordered sensation)
andro-	male	androgens (male hormones)
angio-	blood vessel	angioma (knot of distended blood vessels on the brain)
ante-/ antero-	before, in front	antenatal (before birth)
anti-	against	antipyretic (a drug that reduces fever by lowering the body temperature)
arthro-	joint	arthrotomy (surgical incision of a joint capsule to inspect the contents or drain)
-ary	connected, associated	urinary (associated with urine)
-ase	enzyme	amylase (enzyme concerned with digestion in the breakdown of starch)
bi-/bis-	two	bivalve (consisting of or possessing two valves or sections)
bili-	bile	bilirubin (bile pigment)
bio-	life	biochemistry (the chemistry of life)
bleph-	eyelid	blepharitis (inflammation of the eyelid)
brachi-	arm	brachial artery (an artery of the arm)
brachy-	short	brachydactyly (short fingers or toes)
brady-	slow	bradycardia (abnormally slow heart rate)
broncho-	bronchi	bronchitis (inflammation of the bronchi tubes)
carcino-	cancer	carcinomatosis (carcinoma that has spread widely throughout the body)
cardio-	heart	cardiopathy (any disease of the heart)
carp-/ carpo-	wrist	carpal tunnel syndrome (compression of the median nerve as it enters the palm of the hand)

Component	Meaning	Example
cephal-	head	cephalic (relating to the head)
cerebro-	brain	cerebrospinal fluid (fluid surrounding the brain and spinal cord)
cervic-	cervix/neck	cervicitis (inflammation of the cervix of the uterus)
chemo-	chemical	chemotherapy (treatment to destroy cancerous cells)
cholecyst-	gallbladder	cholecystectomy (surgical removal of the gallbladder)
circum-	around	circumcision (removal of the foreskin around the penis)
coli-	bowel	coliform bacteria (organisms normally found in the gastrointestinal tract)
contra-	against	contraceptive (the prevention of unwanted pregnancy)
cost-	rib	intercostal muscles (muscles between the ribs)
cox-	hip	coxalgia (pain in the hip joint)
crani-	skull	craniotomy (surgical removal of a portion of the skull)
cysto-	bladder	cystoscopy (examination of the urinary bladder by endoscopy)
-cyte	cell	leucocyte (white blood cell)
cyto-	cell	cytology (the study of the structure and function of cells)
de-	away	dehydration (loss or deficiency of water in body tissues)
deci-	tenth	decimal (decimal fraction, a fraction that has a denominator of a power of 10)
demi-, hemi-	half	hemiplegia (paralysis of the arm, leg and trunk on one side of the body)
dent	tooth	dentate (having teeth)
derma-	skin	dermatology (the study of the skin)

(continued)

Component	Meaning	Example
di-/diplo-	two, double	diplopia (double vision)
dis-	separation	dislocation (displacement from their normal position of bones meeting at a joint)
dors-	back	dorsal (relating to the back or posterior part of an organ)
dys-	difficult, painful	dyspnoea (laboured or difficulty breathing)
ec-	out from	ectopic (outside the normal place, such as an embryo developing outside of the uterus)
ecto-	outside	ectopia (misplacement due to either congenital defect or injury of a bodily part)
-ectomy	removal	hysterectomy (removal of the uterus)
electro-	electrical	electrocardiography (technique for recording the electrical activity of the heart)
-emesis	vomiting	hyperemesis (excessive vomiting)
entero-	intestine	enteropathy (disease of the small intestine)
erythr-	red	erythrocyte (red blood cell)
ex-/exo-	away from, out of	extracellular (situated or occurring outside cells)
extra-	outside	extravasation (leakage of blood or fluid from vessels into surrounding tissue)
faci-	face	facial (relating to the face)
ferri-/ferro-	iron	ferrous sulphate (chemical compound used to treat iron deficiency)
feto-/foeto-	fetus/foetus	f(o)etoscopy (inspection of f(o)etus before birth by fibre optics)
galact-	milk	galactorrhoea (abnormally copious milk secretion)
gastr-/gastro-	stomach	gastrin (hormone produced by the stomach)
genito-	genitals	genitourinary (relates to the genital and urinary structures)

Component	Meaning	Example
ger-	old age	gerontology (the study of ageing)
gloss-/ glosso-	tongue	glossitis (inflammation of the tongue)
glyco-	sugar	glycogen (carbohydrate consisting of chains of glucose units)
-gram	a tracing or drawing	electroencephalography (tracing of the brain wave patterns)
-graph	instrument used for recording	electrocardiograph (instrument used for recording heart wave patterns)
gynae-	female	gynaecology (the medical practice dealing with the health of the female reproductive system)
haem-/ haemo-/ haemato-	blood	haemoglobin (red blood cell)
hemi	half	hemianopia (loss of sight in half the visual field)
hepat-/ hepato-	liver	hepatitis (inflammation of the liver)
hetero-	different	heterograft (living tissue graft that is made from one animal species to another)
hist-	tissue	histology (the study of tissue cells)
homeo-	same	homeostasis (physiological process by which internal systems of the body are maintained in equilibrium)
homo-	same	homosexuality (being sexually attracted to member of one's own gender)
hydro-	water	hydropericardium (accumulation of fluid within the membranous sac surrounding the heart)
hygro-	moisture	hygroscopic (having the ability to absorb moisture)
hyper-	above, excessive	hyperglycaemia (an excess of glucose in the bloodstream)
hypno-	sleep	hypnotic (drug which induces sleep)

(continued)

Component	Meaning	Example
hypo	below, deficient	hypothermia (reduction of the body temperature below the normal range)
hyster-	uterus	hysterectomy (the surgical removal of the uterus)
-iasis	condition	parapsoriasis (any one of a group of skin diseases)
-iatrics	healing	geriatrics (branch of medicine that deals with the disorders of later life)
-ician	person skilled in a particular field	physician (registered medical practitioner who specialises in the diagnosis and treatment of disease)
ileo-	ileum	ileostomy (ileum brought through the abdominal wall to create a stoma through which intestinal contents can discharge)
ilio-	ilium	ilium (a wide bone forming the upper part of each side of the hip bone)
im-	not, in	impotent (not potent)
immuno-	immunity	immunosuppressive (a drug that reduces the body's resistance to infection and other foreign bodies by suppressing the immune system)
inter-	between	intercostal muscles (muscles that occupy the spaces between the ribs)
intra-	within	intramuscular (within a muscle)
intro-	inward	introitus (an entrance into a hollow organ or cavity)
-itis	inflammation	appendicitis (infected/inflammed appendix)
lacri-	tears	lacrimation (the production of excess tears)
lact-	milk	lactation (the secretion of milk by the mammary glands)
laparo-	abdomen	lapararotomy (a surgical incision into the abdominal cavity)
laryngo-	larynx	laryngostenosis (narrowing of the cavity of the larynx)

Component	Meaning	Example
later-	side	lateral (situated at or relating to the side)
leuco-/ leuko-	white	leucocytosis (increase in number of leucocytes in the blood)
lip-/lipo-	fat	lipids (fatty substances)
-lysis	breakdown	hydrolysis (breakdown of complex substances by water)
mal-	bad	malnourished (intake of nutrients not enough to sustain good health)
-malacia	softening	osteomalacia (softening of the bones)
mamm-/ mast-	breast	mammogram (radiographic image of the breast)
medi-	middle	median (in the middle – imaginary middle line dividing the body)
mega-/ megalo-	large	megaloblastic (anaemia presenting with abnormally large red cells)
-megaly	enlargement	cardiomegaly (enlarged heart)
melano-	black	melanocytes (skin cells that produce the pigment melanin)
meta-	after, beyond, between	metacarpals (bones situated between the distal row of the carpal bones and the proximal phalanges)
-meter	measure	thermometer (device for measuring temperature)
metro-	uterus	metrorrhagia (bleeding from the uterus other than in the normal menstrual period)
micro-	small	microgram (small unit of measure)
milli-	thousand	millilitre (thousandth part of a litre)
mono-	single, one	monorchism (absence of one testis)
-morph, morpho-	shape, form	morphology (the study of differences in the form between species)
muco-	mucus	mucoid (resembling mucus)
multi-	many	multipara (a woman who has given birth to a live child after each of at least two pregnancies)

(continued)

Component	Meaning	Example
myo-	muscle	myogenic (originating in muscle)
narco-	stupor	narcotic (a drug that induces stupor and is used to relieve pain)
necr-	dead	necrosis (death of tissue)
neo-	new	neonate (an infant during the first four weeks of life)
nephr-/ nephro-	kidney	nephralgia (pain in the kidney, which may be felt in the loin)
neuro-	nerves, nervous system	neurogenic (caused by disease or dysfunction of the nervous system)
noct-	night	nocturia (the passing of urine at night)
oculo-	eye	oculomotor (concerned with eye movements)
odonto-	tooth	odontology (the study of teeth)
oligo-	diminished	oligospermia (the presence of less than the normal number of spermatozoa in the semen)
-ology	science or study of	psychology (the science concerned with the behaviour of human and other animals)
-oma	tumour	glioma (tumour of the glial cells in the nervous system)
onco-	tumour, mass	oncology (the study and practice of treating tumours)
ophthalmo-	eye	ophthalmologist (a doctor who specialises in the diagnosis and treatment of eye diseases)
-opia	defect of vision	hypermetropia (long sight)
orchido-	testis	orchidotomy (incision into the testis, usually performed due to biopsy)
oro-	mouth	oropharynx (the part of the pharynx that lies between the soft palate and the hyoid bone)
orth-	normal, straight	orthodontics (branch of dentistry concerned with growth and development of teeth and the treatment of irregularities)
os-	mouth, bone	ossification (the formation of bone)

Component	Meaning	Example
-osis	condition	osteoporosis (loss of bony tissue resulting in brittle bones)
oss-, osteo-	bone	osteoplasty (plastic surgery of bones)
-ostomy/-stomy	opening	tracheostomy (an opening into the trachea)
ot-/oto-	ear	otorrhagia (bleeding from the ear)
-otomy/-tomy	incision	osteotomy (incision into bone)
ovari-	ovary	ovariotomy (commonly refers to the surgical removal of an ovary)
oxy-	oxygen	oxygenation (the process of becoming saturated with oxygen)
paed-	child	paediatrics (the general medicine of childhood)
para-	beside, near	paramedical (professions closely linked to the medical profession and working in conjunction with them)
part-	birth	parturition (childbirth)
path-	disease	pathological (relating to or arising from disease)
-pathy	disease	nephropathy (kidney disease)
-penia	lack of	leucopenia (lack of white blood cells)
per-	through	perforation (the creation of a hole in an organ, tissue or tube)
peri-	around	pericardium (the membrane surrounding the heart)
perineo-	perineum	perineorrhaphy (surgical repair of a damaged perineum)
-phagia	eating, swallowing	dysphagia (condition in which the act of swallowing may be difficult or painful to perform)
pharmac-	drug	pharmacist (person who is qualified, registered and authorised to dispense drugs)

(continued)

Component	Meaning	Example
pharyngo-	pharynx	pharyngoscope (an endoscope for the examination of the pharynx)
-phasia	speech	aphasia (absence of speech)
phlebo-	vein	phlebotomy (the puncture of a vein in order to withdraw blood)
-phobia/-phobe	fear of	phobia (pathologically strong fear of a particular event or thing, e.g. claustrophobia, the fear of enclosed spaces)
phono-	voice, sound	phonation (the production of sound or voice)
photo-	light	photophobia (an abnormal intolerance of light)
-phylaxis	protection	prophylaxis (a means to prevent disease, such as immunisation)
pilo-	hair	pilonoidal sinus (tract from skin to cleft at the top of the buttocks and containing hairs; the sinus may become infected)
-plasty	reconstruct	rhinoplasty (operation to reconstruct the nose)
-plegia	paralysis	quadriplegia (paralysis affecting all four limbs)
pleur-/pleuro-	pleura	pleurisy (inflammation of the pleura of the lung)
pneumo-	air, lung	pneumothorax (air in the pleural cavity of the lung causing it to collapse)
-pnoea	breathing	dyspnoea (laboured or difficulty breathing)
poly-	many	polydipsia (abnormally intense thirst)
post-	after	post mortem (autopsy)
pre-/pro-	in front, before	premedication (drugs administered to patients before an operation)
pseudo-	false	pseudocyesis (false pregnancy)
psycho-	mind	psychodynamics (the study of the mind)
pulmon-	lung	pulmonary (relating to the lungs)
quadri-	four	quadratus (any four-sided muscle, e.g. femoris, situated at head of femur).

Component	Meaning	Example
radio-	radiation	radio-opaque (having the property of absorbing, and therefore being opaque to X-rays)
retro-	backward	retrograde (going backwards or moving in the opposite direction to normal)
rhin-	nose	rhinitis (inflammation of the mucous membrane of the nose)
-rhythmia	rhythm	arrhythmia (without rhythm; usually applied to a disturbance of the cardiac rhythm)
-rrhage/-rrhagia	to burst, pour	haemorrhage (the escape of blood from a blood vessel)
-rrhoea	flow, discharge	leucorrhoea (white, vaginal discharge)
sacro-	sacrum	sacrococcygeal (relating to or between the sacrum and the coccyx)
-scope	instrument for examining	otoscope (apparatus used for examining the eardrum and external meatus)
-scopy	to examine, looking	gastroscopy (endoscopic examination of the stomach)
semi-	half	semicircular canals (three tubes that form part of the membranous labyrinth of the ear)
somni-	sleep	insomnia (unable to sleep)
-sonic	sound	ultrasonic (high frequency sound beyond the sound of the human ear)
sphygm-	pulse	sphygmomanometer (instrument for measuring arterial blood pressure)
splen-/spleno-	spleen	splenectomy (surgical removal of the spleen)
spondyl-/spondylo-	vertebra	spondylolisthesis (forward shift of vertebra upon each other due to defect in the joints)
-stasis	stand still, lack of movement	haemostasis (no bleeding)
steno-	narrow	stenostomia (the abnormal narrowing of an opening)

(continued)

Component	Meaning	Example
stern-/ sterno-	sternum	sternocleidomastoid muscle (muscle that extends from the mastoid process (in the neck) to he sternum and clavicle)
super-/ supra-	above	suprapubic (above the pubic bone)
tachy-	fast	tachycardia (an increase in heart rate above normal)
tars-/tarso-	foot, eyelid	tarsalgia (aching pain arising from the tarsus in the foot)
tetra-	four	tetradactyly (congenital abnormally in which there are only four digits on a hand or a foot)
thermo-	heat, temperature	thermoreceptor (sensory nerve ending that responds to heat or to cold)
thorac-/ thoraco-	chest	thoracoplasty (surgical repair of abnormalities or defects of the thorax)
throm-/ thrombo-	clot	thrombocyte (platelet)
thyro-	thyroid	thyroglossal (relating to the thyroid gland and tongue)
tox-	poison	toxicology (the study of poisonous materials and their effects on living organisms)
trache-/ trachea-	trachea	tracheostomy (surgical operation to form a hole in the trachea; a tube is then placed into this hole)
trans-	across, through	transection (a cross-section of a piece of tissue)
tri-	three	tridactyly (congenital abnormality in which there are only three digits on a hand or foot)
trich-	hair	trichomycosis (any hair disease caused by an infection with a fungus)
ultra-	beyond, extreme	ultrasonics (the study of uses and properties of ultrasound)
uni-	one	unilateral (relating to or affecting one side of the body)

Component	Meaning	Example
uretero-	ureter	ureterocele (a cystic swelling of the wall of the ureter at the point where it passes into the bladder)
urethr-/ urethra-	urethra	urethritis (inflammation of the urethra)
uri-/uro-	urine	urinometer (a hydrometer for measuring the specific gravity of the urine)
-uria	urine	dysuria (pain or difficulty passing urine)
vas-/vaso-	vessel, duct	vascular (relating to or supplied with blood vessels)
vene-	vein	venepuncture (the puncture of a vein to withdraw blood for laboratory testing)
viscer-	organs	visceroptosis (the downward displacement of the abdominal organs)
xero-	dry	xeroderma (dry skin)
zoo-	animal	zoonosis (an infectious disease of animals that can be transmitted to humans, e.g. rabies)

Appendix 2

WEIGHT CONVERSION CHARTS

Care Skills for Nurses, First Edition. Claire Boyd
© 2014 John Wiley & Sons, Ltd. Published 2014 by John Wiley & Sons, Ltd.

KILOGRAMS TO POUNDS

1 kg = 2.2 lb

kg	lb	kg	lb	kg	lb	kg	lb	kg	lb	kg	lb
1	2.2	21	46.2	41	90.2	61	134.2	81	178.2	101	222.2
2	4.4	22	48.4	42	92.4	62	136.4	82	180.4	102	224.4
3	6.6	23	50.6	43	94.6	63	138.6	83	182.6	103	226.6
4	8.8	24	52.8	44	96.8	64	140.8	84	184.8	104	228.8
5	1.0	25	55.0	45	99.0	65	143.0	85	187.0	105	231.0
6	13.2	26	57.2	46	101.2	66	145.2	85	189.2	106	233.3
7	15.4	27	59.4	47	103.4	67	147.4	87	191.4	107	235.4
8	17.6	28	61.6	48	105.6	68	149.6	88	193.6	108	237.6
9	19.8	29	63.8	49	107.8	69	151.8	89	195.8	109	239.8
10	22.0	30	66.0	50	110.0	70	154.0	90	198.0	110	242.0
11	24.2	31	68.2	51	112.2	71	156.2	91	200.2	111	244.2
12	26.4	32	70.4	52	114.4	72	158.4	92	202.4	112	246.4
13	28.6	33	72.6	53	116.6	73	160.6	93	204.6	113	248.6
14	30.8	34	74.8	54	118.8	74	162.8	94	206.8	114	250.8
15	33.0	35	77.0	55	121.0	75	165.0	95	209.0	115	253.0
16	35.2	36	79.2	56	123.2	76	167.2	96	211.2	116	255.2
17	37.4	37	81.4	57	125.4	77	169.4	97	213.4	117	257.4
18	39.6	38	83.6	58	127.6	78	171.6	98	215.6	118	259.6
19	41.8	39	85.8	59	129.8	79	173.8	99	217.8	119	261.8
20	44.0	40	88.0	60	132.0	80	176.0	100	220.0	120	264.0

STONES TO KILOGRAMS

1 stone = 6.35 kg

stones	kg	stones	kg
1	6.35	15	95.25
2	12.7	16	101.6
3	19.05	17	107.95
4	25.4	18	114.3
5	31.75	19	120.65
6	38.1	20	127.0
7	44.45	21	133.35
8	50.8	22	139.7
9	57.15	23	146.05
10	63.5	24	152.4
11	69.85	25	158.75
12	76.2	26	165.1
13	82.55	27	171.45
14	88.9	28	177.8

POUNDS TO KILOGRAMS

1 lb = 0.45 kg

lb	kg
1	0.45
2	0.9
3	1.35
4	1.8
5	2.25
6	2.7
7	3.15
8	3.6
9	4.05
10	4.5
11	4.95
12	5.4
13	5.85
14 (1 stone)	6.35

Index

Care Skills for Nurses, First Edition. Claire Boyd
© 2014 John Wiley & Sons, Ltd. Published 2014 by John Wiley & Sons, Ltd.

Printed and bound by CPI Group (UK) Ltd, Croydon, CR0 4YY
09/08/2021

03078578-0001